OCCUPATIONAL THERAPY FOR CHILDREN WITH DISABILITIES

THERAPY IN PRACTICE
Series Editor: Jo Campling

This series of books is aimed at 'therapists' concerned with rehabilitation in a very broad sense. The intended audience particularly includes occupational therapists, physiotherapists and speech therapists, but many titles will also be of interest to nurses, psychologists, medical staff, social workers, teachers or volunteer workers. Some volumes will be interdisciplinary, others aimed at one particular profession. All titles will be comprehensive but concise, and practical but with due reference to relevant theory and evidence. They are not research monographs but focus on professional practice, and will be of value to both students and qualified personnel.

Titles Available

Living Skills for Mentally Handicapped People
Christine Peck and Chia Swee Hong

Communication Problems in Elderly People
Rosemary Gravell

Rehabilitation of the Severely Brain-Injured Adult
Edited by Ian Fussey and Gordon Muir Giles

Physiotherapy and the Elderly Patient
Paul Wagstaff and Davis Coakley

Titles in Preparation

Modern Electrotherapy
Christopher Hayne

Assessment of Physically Disabled People at Home
Kathleen Maczka

Occupational Therapy Practice in Psychiatry
Linda Finlay

Movement Exercises for Language Difficulties
M. Nash-Wortham

Management in Occupational Therapy
Zielfa B. Maslin

Community Occupational Therapy with Mentally Handicapped People
Debbie Isaac

Understanding Dysphasia
Lesley Jordan and Rita Twiston Davies

Psychology in Physiotherapy
Cynthia Fox

Working with Bilingual Language Disability
Edited by Deirdre M. Duncan

Rehabilitation of the Older Patient
Edited by Amanda J. Squires

Dysarthria: Theory and Therapy
Sandra J. Robertson

Occupational Therapy for the Brain-injured Adult
Jo Clark-Wilson and Gordon Muir Giles

Speech and Language Problems in Children
Dilys A. Treharne

Therapy in the Treatment of Early Head-injured Patients
Ruth Garner

Occupational Therapy for Children with Disabilities

DOROTHY E. PENSO
Senior Occupational Therapist,
Child Development Centre,
York District Hospital

Illustrations by TERRY WINSTON

CROOM HELM
London & Sydney

Croom Helm Ltd, Provident House,
Burrell Row, Beckenham, Kent BR3 1AT
Croom Helm Australia, 44–50 Waterloo Road,
North Ryde, 2113, New South Wales

British Library Cataloguing in Publication Data

Penso, Dorothy E.
Occupational therapy for children with disabilities.
1. Occupational therapy for children
2. Handicapped children — Care and treatment
I. Title
615.8'5152 RJ53.025

ISBN 0–7099–4049–1

Photosetting by Mayhew Typesetting, Bristol, England
Printed and bound in Great Britain by Mackays of Chatham Ltd, Kent

Contents

Acknowledgements

During the last 14 years I have learned more from the hundreds of children with impairments I have met than I have been able to teach them. Their parents have taught me which strategies are effective and which are not. Children, mothers, fathers, thank you. I also appreciate the help and support I have received, especially in preparing this manuscript, from the paediatric team of which I am a member. I thank Eileen Winterbottom, Head Occupational Therapist, for reading, correcting and commenting on the text and Jo Campling, Editor, for her support and encouragement. I appreciate the practical support and patience of my husband, Giovanni, during the many months in which I have been preoccupied with the manuscript.

Note

Throughout the text the pronoun 'he' refers to the child and 'she' to the therapist, in order to avoid any confusion which may arise by the use of 'he/she' or 's/he'. There are, of course, both male and female therapists and both girls and boys suffer from impairments; however, there are more women than men in the therapeutic professions and a higher percentage of boys than girls suffer from continuing impairment.

Introduction

Occupational therapists who work in the field of paediatrics will meet children who suffer from a vast range of both congenital and acquired impairments. These impairments may give rise to disabilities which severely restrict the lifestyle of the child and his family or they may, to the untrained observer, appear to be almost negligible. Impairments may arise from neurological deficits such as cerebral palsy, metabolic abnormalities, such as the mucopolysaccharidoses, infections such as meningitis, trauma as in road traffic accidents (RTA), or genetic anomalies which may be inherited or arise from a mutation as in one type of Down's Syndrome.

Impairments of childhood may have physical manifestations only, or, in addition, there may be mental involvement which affects intellectual achievement, the child's emotional stability and his capacity to perform the activities of daily living. In other children mental incapacity may predominate with perhaps minor physical symptoms. Few children have a single disability, most have a number of impairments which affect more than one facet of life. For example, some children who suffer from one of the forms of cerebral palsy may in addition to their physical disability have poor intellectual abilities and emotional problems; a considerable percentage, 30 per cent (Fisch, 1969), of those who suffer from athetoid cerebral palsy have a high frequency hearing loss.

Spina bifida has many physical manifestations: in addition to the obvious lack of movement and sensation below the level of the lesion, bowel and bladder involvement, spinal and lower limb deformities are frequently seen. These children may also have significant perceptual difficulties, language problems which may not be immediately apparent and fine motor deficit which is often first noticed when the child experiences difficulty with handwriting during his first years in school.

Children who some would describe as 'clumsy' but are more kindly said 'to lack grace', may have difficulties which are of a sensory, perceptual or motor nature, though more commonly these difficulties arise from a combination of causes. Those who suffer from juvenile chronic arthritis (JCA) often have severe problems with poor self-image and peer relationships.

It would be a daunting, if not impossible, task to set down in one volume the total impairments which affect children together with suggestions for suitable occupational therapy techniques, equipment and toys. Such a volume would be repetitious and the emphasis would be on the impairment rather than the whole child and his family. Each child is unique and although two may have the same clinical diagnosis their treatments differ because of the personality of the child, and the philosophy, lifestyle and expectations of his family.

There are many books available, some of which are referred to in the text or listed in the further reading section, which describe the clinical aspects of the impairments of childhood. Manufacturers' and distributors' catalogues are freely available and occupational therapists are able to build up their own library of sources of equipment and toys.

This book, therefore, attempts to look deeper and beyond individual impairments to the basic approach of the occupational therapist to the child with disabilities and his family. It considers the child's environment, his family and his therapists as transmitters of appropriate stimuli to which he will react with appropriate behaviour and thus learn, the barriers which may impede the transmission of those stimuli, the child's reception and perception of them and his response to them. In later chapters assessment and treatment are discussed based on defining and solving problems relevant to the life of a particular child and his family. It provides a basis of paediatric occupational therapy for students and occupational therapists beginning to specialise in this field.

1

Children and Parents, Therapists and Impairment

Childhood is not only a preparation for later life and adulthood: it is life.
Professor Jack Tizzard

NORMAL CHILDHOOD

Learning about the world begins at the moment of birth, some would even assert before birth, when the child experiences sensations from his environment and the people and objects within it. He begins to accumulate memories of experiences on which he will draw in the future. He moves within his limited world in response to sensory stimulation which he perceives or processes and thus learns to adapt to his surroundings. As a result of neurological maturation and practice the child's range of motor skills becomes more extensive and complex, sensory experience widens and his perceptions of his world become more meaningful.

His methods of locomotion become increasingly sophisticated until he is able to walk, run, climb and balance on a very narrow base. His manipulative skills mature until he is able to locate accurately the tiniest objects, pick them up, place and release them using a precise index finger and thumb grip. He learns to manipulate objects so that he may examine their structure, shape, size, weight, colour and texture.

With repetition he begins to make sense of the sound systems — language — with which people communicate. He understands complex sentences which contain a number of elements. He practises using words himself and becomes increasingly skilful at making his needs known verbally. As his ability to use the symbolism of words increases, he becomes skilled at talking about things which are not present in his environment, events which have taken place in the past and those which are anticipated in the future.

With the addition of verbal symbolism he makes sense of concepts such as, same and different, bigger than and smaller than, the relationship of objects to each other and to himself, in front, behind, beside, above and below. He begins to understand speed and distance in relation to himself and between other objects and people.

Parents

The child is more than a phenomenal learning machine, he is a person, who has his own unique personality and perception of the world. Parents are proud of each step towards independence which their child takes, his first smile, the first time he sits without support, his first broad-based steps. Parenthood is also fraught with difficulties, sleepless nights, periods of negative behaviour, temper tantrums and sibling jealousy.

Most parents are anxious to provide their child with play materials which they believe will encourage the development of new skills. They provide situations which will enlarge their child's experience and knowledge yet when the vast amount of learning takes place in the first few years of life is considered it becomes apparent that much of this learning is accomplished entirely by the child when the required level of neurological maturation has been reached. No child will walk in a normal fashion until his nervous system has reached the appropriate level of maturation. It would be difficult for a child to understand the qualities of heat and cold without having the sensory channels to experience it. Except those deprived of even the most basic experiences, children learn for themselves many of the skills and much of the knowledge which is necessary to adapt and survive.

Most children, regardless of their parents' attitudes and child rearing practices, will indicate the direction in which their interests lie. Parental encouragement moves along parallel with the interests of their child. A child who has just perfected, at about two and a half years, the skill of jumping with two feet together will spend many hours perfecting the movement. A child whose current interest is words will engage his parents in endless dialogue and probably demand their time and attention for story telling and reading.

Parents and children progress along a mutual path of discovery, learning and skill acquisition. Most who follow the path do so with a fair degree of success. It is almost as if parent and child possess some foreknowledge of this previously untrod path of parenthood and childhood.

Is the same path followed by the family and the child who has one or more disabilities?

PARENTS WHO HAVE CHILDREN WITH IMPAIRMENTS

Frequently in the moments following childbirth, a mother's first question to the staff in attendance is, 'Is the baby all right?' Parents expect, for nine months, a perfect child, a child who has the potential to grow into a physically, mentally and emotionally normal person. Should a child be born with an impairment which is apparent at the moment of birth, parents are deeply shocked and experience a period of mourning for the 'death' of the perfect child which they expected. They may initially experience feelings of rejection towards their child which may later be replaced by overwhelming desires to protect their especially vulnerable child. Parents may refuse to accept the gravity of the disability or feel, perhaps unrealistically, that it will go away. Parents may deny that they have ever been told certain facts because at the time they were not receptive to them. There are likely to be times when parents attempt to apportion blame for their child's disability. They will search their minds for events or actions prior to their child's birth which could have caused the imperfection. They may feel that they caused their child's disability by something they did or failed to do. Each parent may look for the cause of the disability in the other or the other's family. The birth of a child who has a disability is often a complicated one and parents may blame the staff in attendance at the birth for their child's condition. They may cite the inadequacy of the equipment available, lack of attention or mishandling of the birth.

At some point most parents recognise the disability and do all in their power to help their child make the most of his assets and where possible overcome or find ways to bypass the problem. Most parents learn to cope for the present, unlike professionals who have had experience of many children with disabling conditions and are aware of the likely course the child's and his parents' life will take.

The birth of a child must, necessarily, alter the dynamics within the family. The birth, especially of the first child often has a drastic effect on the relationship between the mother and the father — for the first time there is another person to consider besides themselves.

One of the partners may give up paid employment to care for the infant and, therefore, that partner's contact with the outside world may become very sparse. There is often a reduction in the income of the couple with a young child. Future children born into the family again alter its dynamics; there is usually sibling rivalry of some kind, family income will be required to stretch still further, the mother and father will have even less time to spend alone with each other.

Whatever potential abilities or disabilities a child is born with, he is first their child, not a disabled child. He is a child who has the same needs for care and love as other children, who has similar effects on the nuclear and extended family as any other child. He may also have special needs peculiar to his disabilities. His problems will create special needs within the family.

He is likely to need more care and attention than an able child. He may require frequent feeds, his meal times may be protracted. There are times when most children have disturbed sleeping patterns, but the child with a disability may never sleep through the night, requiring parental attention at frequent intervals with the result that it becomes difficult for parents to cope with his day time demands and those of his siblings. There may be a need, especially in the early years, for frequent hospital visits for medical attention and sessions with a variety of therapists. Such visits are expensive both in time and money and can strain the physical, emotional and financial resources of the family.

Many disabilities, of course, are not apparent at birth. It may be some time before the milder forms of conditions such as cerebral palsy, mental handicap and visual or auditory impairment are diagnosed. Many children have to spend a number of terms in school before it is appreciated that they suffer from specific learning difficulties. Other continuing disabilities such as juvenile chronic arthritis (JCA) are not present at birth but develop during childhood. Parents of such children experience many of the same emotional and physical problems as those whose children's disability was manifest at birth.

Impairment

Childhood is a time of increasing ability, extending experience and boundless curiosity. Is life equally full of newness for the child who is born with or acquires an impairment? The answer does not depend entirely on the severity of the impairment but on how that impairment affects the child's ability to exchange information with the physical world and in social interactions (Fraser, 1980). The child who suffers from athetosis will receive less information from his environment because of his poor skills of manipulation compared with the unimpaired child. He may also suffer from a high frequency hearing loss which will reduce his auditory input and also impair his ability to communicate verbally with others. Such a child will suffer from limitation of experience and a paucity of stimulation which may be more significant reasons for impairment to his development and life skills than his athetosis.

A second factor is that, generally, the world is organised to suit the needs of the non-impaired. This organisation differs in various parts of the world in that an impairment which is significant in one culture or era passes unnoticed in a different area or age. At a meeting of the British Paediatric Association in York a few years ago, Dr Martin Bax described an impairment which was prevalent in ancient Greece; it affected only males, mainly sons of noble families and greatly restricted their ability to function successfully within their environment. Fortunately it is rarely diagnosed today. Its most significant symptom was the inability to use a sword! (Penso, 1981). Dr Bax's anecdote illustrates very succinctly how various impairments may be of greater or lesser significance depending on time and place.

The third factor is attitude towards the impaired child (Fraser, 1980). Most children who suffer from impairment are investigated in a medical setting. The child with mental impairment will in many instances undergo clinical tests to investigate the reasons for his intellectual incapacity. The child with visual impairment will be seen by an ophthalmologist, perhaps a paediatrician and an orthoptist usually in a hospital setting which by its nature suggests sickness to both the child and his parents. Though the child is not sick it is very easy for the family to adopt the same attitude towards the child as they would towards a sick person. Traditionally the sick are absolved from many of life's responsibilities; it is so easy to give the same dispensations to the child with impairment with dire results on his development and self-expectations.

Looking at impairment from these points of view illustrates the implications of the brief definition of impairment provided by the World Health Organization: 'Any loss or abnormality of psychological, physiological of anatomical structure or function' (Wood, 1980).

Disability

Impairments do not necessarily become disabilities although many of them are likely to do so. The absence of a little finger mars the completeness of the hand as does the absence of a thumb. The former is an impairment, the latter an impairment and a disability. From a functional point of view, except for people such as pianists or typists, the little finger plays only a minor role in hand function and even such people would after a time successfully adapt to the loss. The thumb and its apposition to the fingers, however, plays a vital part in most fine motor skills and its loss, particularly from the preferred hand, is a major disability. Cerebral palsy may prevent a pupil recording his work with a pen or pencil in school; however, it does not preclude the recording of the same information on a typewriter or electronic printer. Such a child has an impairment — the lack of fine motor control; he also has disability — lack of the effective control of a pen or pencil necessary to write. This impairment and disability need not be handicapping.

When considering disabilities the problems are related directly to the person, whereas impairment relates to the medical model of observed manifestation of pathology. The term disability relates to performance and activity, its definition describes the effect of impairment in relation to the lifestyle of the person who suffers from a disability. It may be defined as 'any restriction or lack (resulting from an impairment) of ability to perform an activity in the manner or within the range considered normal for a human being' (Wood, 1980).

It may be suggested that the child has only ever known himself as he is, for he perceives himself as 'normal' until others notice and remark upon his impairment and then treat him differently from his unimpaired peers. Kashani (1986) describes a five-year-old girl with unilateral facial paralysis who came home from nursery school and complained to her mother that the other children were laughing at her. She had seen her own reflection in the mirror daily without undue concern. It was the reaction of others to her impairment which affected her self-concept.

It may be some time before a child realises that he lacks abilities which are common to his peer group and frequently that realisation is precipitated by the responses of peers, parents and other adults. Disability in childhood must also be balanced against the child's development level. An impairment may only become a disability if it restricts performance of activities which are considered normal at that stage of development. Cerebral palsy may prevent a child of one year from using a precise finger thumb grip to pick up crumbs of food: this impairment of function is a disability since an able one-year-old child would frequently indulge in such an activity. That same impairment of function would, theoretically, prevent the child holding a lace in order to thread beads but at one year of age this is not a disability for the child because, developmentally, children of this age are not able to thread beads. Disability in childhood must always consider impairment of function together with the expected developmental level.

Handicap

An impairment or disability may become a handicap though the aims, particularly with children, are to prevent as far as possible the development of handicap if the World Health Organisation's definition is accepted: 'Handicap: a disadvantage for a given individual, resulting from an impairment or a disability, that limits or prevents the fulfilment of a role that is normal (depending on age, sex, and social and cultural factors) for that individual' (Wood, 1980). A child has potential for development, maturation and the capacity to devise alternative methods of function. He has not yet decided his own lifestyle, occupation or means of economic self-sufficiency.

It is with disability that occupational therapists are chiefly concerned, for they are 'enablers' who devise means by which the child may function within his environment. 'Enabling' will include the active participation of the child in developing his capacities to the maximum level possible and the provision of equipment and devices to help the child attain optimum independence in the areas of communication, personal care appropriate to his developmental age, gross and fine movement, appropriate body posture and skills suitable to his lifestyle.

Table 1.1 shows some of the conditions of childhood with the range of disabilities that may accompany them.

THE ROLE OF THE OCCUPATIONAL THERAPIST IN PAEDIATRICS

Occupational therapy is always based on *purposeful* activity, which

Table 1.1: Some conditions of childhood and some of the disabilities which *may* occur in them

Condition	Disability			
	Motor	Sensory	Cerebral	Behavioural
Cerebral Palsy	Spasticity Athetosis Hemiplegia Diplegia Athetosis	Visual impairment Impaired hearing Visual field defect Occasionally deafness High frequency hearing loss	Limited intelligence Perceptual difficulties	
	Ataxia		Limited intelligence	
Spina bifida	Paralysis below level of lesion Fine motor deficit	Loss of tactile sensation below level of lesion Frequently visual impairment, particularly nystagmus	Frequently below average inteligence Poor comprehension of language Perceptual difficulties	Poor motivation
Head injury	Symptoms of neurological trauma	Visual impairment temporary/permanent	Receptive, expressive language impairment depending on site of injury Poor concentration Amnesia Temporary/permanent intellectual deficit	Depression Emotional liability Personality change Psychiatric disturbance

Muscular dystrophy	Muscle weakness	—	Average IQ 80–85	Problems associated with degenerative condition
Arthrogryposis neuropathic, myopathic	Joint limitation Fixed extension Muscle weakness Flexion contractures	—	—	—
Juvenile chronic arthritis	Pain, stiffness Limited range of movement	—	—	Poor self-esteem Poor peer relationships
Down's syndrome	Hypotonia Joint laxity	—	Mental handicap Poor language development	—
Specific learning problems	Poor coordination Dyspraxia	Sometimes visual problems Sometimes minor hearing problems	Perceptual problems Poor body image Spatial difficulties	Compensation by withdrawal or attention seeking behaviour
Mental handicap	Poor coordination and balance Poor motor planning Sometimes very agile	Hearing and/or visual deficits	Low IQ Perceptual difficulties Epilepsy	Behaviour problems Ritualistic activity

Table 1.1 *contd.*

Condition	Disability			
	Motor	Sensory	Cerebral	Behavioural
Morquio's syndrome	Joint deformity and limitation Limited mobility	—	—	Poor self-esteem Poor peer relationships
Dystonia musculorum deformans	Increasing dystonia Swallowing difficulties Articulation difficulties	—	—	Depression Poor self-esteem
Prader-Willi syndrome	Hypotonia poor sucking and feeding, motor delay	50% decreased pain sensation	IQ moderate impairment/low normal	—
Tuberose sclerosis	—	retinal lesions	Seizures Intellectual impairment variable	—
Congenital rubella	Spastic diplegia	Deafness Cataract Microphthalmia Congenital glaucoma Retinopathy	Poor language acquisition out of proportion with deafness Low IQ	Sometimes autistic behaviour patterns
Hypothyroidism	Abnormal gait, tremor ataxia	—	Mental impairment Learning disabilities	—

is relevant to the client's lifestyle, physical and mental capacities and his disability. Occupational therapy has been described as: 'The treatment of physical and psychiatric conditions through specific activities in order to help people reach their maximum level of function and independence in all aspects of family life' (British Association of Occupational Therapists, 1982). Occupational therapists entering the speciality of paediatrics will, of course, need to undertake further study and observation in order to become proficient. They must study the medical aspects of the disabilities of childhood and learn assessment and treatment techniques. The occupational therapist's knowledge of self-help equipment and adaptations must be augmented to include those specific to children.

She must be able to assess the child's current developmental level in order to help him progress successfully to the next stage. The aims and behavioural objectives for a particular child will not only be based upon his current developmental level but also upon his *rate* of development. Behavioural objectives will be planned so that the child is successful and thus be motivated to further effort.

The occupational therapist will look at the child's specific impairments in relation to his daily life and devise methods to overcome or circumvent difficulties. She will provide self-help equipment, commercially available or custom-made, which enables him to function at his developmental level. It should be kept to the minimum necessary to facilitate function always bearing in mind the child's developmental potential and the fact that equipment may outlive its usefulness. Special equipment always suggests inability and its provision must always be weighed against the child's potential for development and ability to discover his own methods of accomplishing tasks.

The occupational therapist will know that childhood is a time of continual learning, and her plans will include maximum opportunity for discovery and the satisfaction of curiosity. Broadly, the child's life consists of activities in the home including the gradual acquisition of self-care skills, play in its widest sense (not necessarily only with conventional toys) and later, activities at nursery and school. For the severely impaired child a proportion of occupational therapy will be directed towards the parents or carers to advise on handling techniques and the best methods of carrying out the child's daily care.

A further area in which occupational therapy is important is the assessment of function; this may be necessary, for example, during a drug trial when specific evidence is being sought regarding its effect on the child. Similar testing may be necessary when it is suspected that the child is suffering from a degenerative condition. Tests must be devised which are valid, i.e. they test what they purport to test, and reliable, i.e. it must be possible to replicate them on a number of occasions (Vernon, 1960, pp. 45–8).

The occupational therapist enabling others to handle the child therapeutically

No therapist can work with children without positive communication with others concerned with the child. Unlike adults, children cannot live independently; they need the love and care of parents or parent substitutes. Many children have siblings and an extended family who are concerned with the child's progress and achievements, his limitations and failures. Formal therapy takes up a comparatively small proportion of a child's life, particularly in his early years. Most time is spent at home and parents and family can become his most effective therapists if treatment aims and behavioural objects are explained and demonstrated to them.

It may be easier to exclude others from formal therapy sessions, because the child may concentrate on an activity for longer periods and he will have no opportunity to play one adult off against another. The therapist will be able to give her complete attention to the child and she may feel that she can handle the child more appropriately without other members of his family present. Such a therapy session will be an isolated experience for the child which bears little relation to his real life situation. Therapy which includes the observations, questions and comments of parents is, in most cases, likely to be carried over into the home situation, where it will become meaningful, realistic and frequently practised. Explanations, however explicit, of unseen treatment are not adequate substitutes for active participation and demonstration of effect.

As children become older their world enlarges, many attend day nurseries and later school. Occupational therapists have a number of unique skills which they must share with nursery staff and teachers if children who have disabilities are to be given the greatest opportunities to attain their maximum potential.

Occupational therapy can improve all aspects of childhood by facilitating self-care at a level appropriate to the child's physical abilities and mental development, by devising and adapting play material to promote symbolic, imaginative, cognitive constructional and manual skills and by suggesting suitable equipment to facilitate formal education. It will also enable the child to demonstrate that he has learned.

The occupational therapist and the therapeutic team

Most children require the expertise of various disciplines. It is essential that they communicate one with another to attain economy of effort and to ensure that conflicting advice is not reaching those who care for the child. In order to communicate effectively it is necessary for each discipline to understand something of the others' expertise.

The exact manner in which therapists work together will vary according to the type of establishment in which they work. Three types of developmental paediatric teams have been described (Cotton, 1984). 'The MDT (multi-disciplinary team) is based on friendly co-operation amongst various professionals.' Therapists are based within the same building but each conducts her own assessment and treatment, meeting together to discuss their several assessments, treatments and progress. 'The IDT (inter-disciplinary team) is a forward looking team, closely knit and *goal directed.*' Such a team will work together to devise a collective treatment plan for a particular child, making an overall plan of aims and behavioural objectives so that the child and his parents may be presented with one plan of treatment. 'The TDT (trans-disciplinary team), like the IDT, is goal directed and also based on integrating expertise, but the TDT aims at a further step in integration, one where any member of the team will be able to do another person's job so that the most suitable worker can be chosen to deal with a specific child.'

Other members of the paediatric team

The paediatrician is a doctor who has specialised in the diseases of childhood. Some specialise still further and become experts in neonatal medicine, others are experts in the acute diseases of childhood or in child neurology or chronic disabilities. The paediatrician is usually the leader of the team of experts concerned with the child, co-ordinating information from team members to provide a complete picture of the child and his strengths and weaknesses.

Impairment has already been described as a medical model and it is from this angle that the paediatrician initially will view the child, noting loss or abnormality of structure or function. From these facts it may be possible to arrive at a diagnosis, prognosis and medical treatment for the condition although in many impairments of childhood this may not be possible.

Hearing tests are taken by a variety of specialists, by audiologists and audiometricians. A doctor experienced with children and who has undertaken special study of audiometry in relation to children with multiple impairments might also administer hearing tests. The skills required are more complex than those of the testing of hearing in an able child; if hearing is one of a number of impairments in a child the tester needs skills in interpreting the responses when there is motor and/or language impairment.

Hearing loss is described in terms of frequency, the pitch of sounds which the child is able to hear, and the volume of sound necessary for the child to hear measured in decibels. Both these qualities are usually recorded in graph form which illustrates the strengths and weaknesses of the child's hearing.

Free field testing may be used with babies: the infant is seated on the lap of his mother or another adult whilst a second adult attracts his attention with a soundless toy. His hearing is then measured by a third person who makes sounds, out of sight of the child, to his left and to his right. The Stycar Test (Sheridan, 1968) uses the human voice, a high frequency rattle, a spoon stirred round a cup, crumpling paper and a bell. The very young baby will 'still' when he hears a new sound and the older one will turn towards the sound.

This type of testing allows an estimate of the child's level of hearing to be made but it does not provide a precise assessment. With the multiply impaired child who cannot indicate when he has heard a sound it may be necessary to condition him to make some observable response to the sounds of various pitches and levels transmitted to him through earphones from an audiometer. The occupational therapist will be able to devise special toys or equipment to be used by the severely impaired child so that he will make reliable responses.

The orthoptist is an expert in the use of vision. A child may have a level of visual acuity adequate for his lifestyle but he may not be making the best use of it because of other visual impairments; for example, the inability to use both eyes together which would result in diplopia (double vision) or lack of stereopsis (depth perception). Orthoptists assess how eyesight is used and treat diagnosed defects. They are mainly concerned with defective binocular vision and abnormal eye movements.

The orthoptist, who works with the ophthalmic surgeon, may be hospital based or she may work in the community on screening programmes. Orthoptists use standardised tests such as the Snellen chart and Stycar Tests to assess vision, so young children who could not co-operate in adult tests are able to have accurate assessments made of how they are using their eyes.

Many orthoptists work with children who have additional physical and/or mental impairments with whom it is not possible to use standard tests and ingenious methods have been evolved to test the use of vision of such children.

The physiotherapist is an expert in helping children to attain their potential independent movement and to attain and maintain posture. She will assess the child's current level of physical development in relation to his ability to attain and maintain postures and movements appropriate to the activities he will undertake at his developmental level. This will include the type, strength and distribution of his muscle tone which is particularly significant where spasticity, hypotonia or ataxia is present. She will observe his modes of locomotion again in relation to the methods most usually employed by a child at his developmental level. She will note any abnormal patterns of movement, the presence or absence of righting and balance reactions and the presence of or the likelihood of the development of contractures and deformities.

The methods she will use to treat these impairments will depend upon the specialist training she has undertaken and her personal philosophy which has evolved from that training. A large proportion of her time will be spent with the child and his parents, demonstrating to the latter how to handle their child at home during daily living activities as well as home treatment sessions.

Depending upon the developmental age of the child and the nature of his impairments the physiotherapist may treat children individually or in groups. Children suffering from JCA are an example of those who benefit particularly from the friendly competition of a group setting.

The speech therapist is concerned with all aspects of language and pathology. Many speech therapists work exclusively with children and they are experts in the stages of language development from infancy when the baby begins to make babbling sounds to late childhood when the comprehension and expression of a large vocabulary, complex syntax and the articulation of all the phenomena within a language have been mastered.

Speech therapy includes the use of standardised tests which are used to assess the child's level of understanding of what is said to him and the developmental level at which he is able to express himself. Both of these types of test may have elements which allow the speech therapist to assess the size of his vocabulary, use of phrases and sentences. Other tests may analyse a child's ability to vocalise specific speech sounds. Using such tests and her own experience the speech therapist will be able to decide on the nature of a child's difficulties, whether his problem is one of developmental delay or deviant development of language.

Speech therapists are concerned with the assessment of children whose hearing is impaired and the selection of suitable means of communication. Non-verbal means of communication are not, however, only taught to children who have impaired hearing but also to some who have autistic symptoms, or to children who have a mental handicap and retardation of language development.

Many children lack the physical ability to make signs effectively with their hands. It may be decided that such a child would benefit from one of the communication systems which relies on the selection of words, symbols or pictures which are suitably arranged on a board or from an electronic display (Heddell, 1985, pp. 15-24).

The nurse today usually bases her approach on the 'nursing process' which is patient orientated and geared towards problem solving. 'This standard method of problem solving includes the following steps:

observing and recognising the problem;
defining the problem;
arriving at possible solutions to the problem;
putting those solutions to work;
determining if those solutions have been successful' (Butts, 1980).

'Nurses apply the nursing process and record it by means of "problem orientated medical records" (POMR) of which there are five components: data base or initial assessment; problem list; initial plan; progress notes; and discharge summary' (Vasey, 1980). Establishments which adopt such records will, of course, require occupational therapists to integrate their records.

The nursing process and POMR are particularly suited to paediatric nursing where not only the child's problems but also those of his family must be considered. Nursing which considers a child's usual sleeping pattern, his eating habits, his preferred types of play and the like will be effective.

When a child enters hospital with an acute illness he does so because at that time the child needs care which the family cannot give. Many paediatric nurses see themselves as 'enablers' in the sense that they make it possible for the parents to cope with their sick child. Nurses undertake the medical care of children and in some cases teach parents how to administer that care. The nurse does not attempt to remove the care of the child from his parents; in many cases she has much to learn from them. A very wise nursing sister has said of parents, 'Nurses have more to learn than to teach'.

Children with continuing disability also have acute illnesses or require medical investigations which require hospital admissions. On these occasions the occupational therapist has the opportunity to work together with the ward staff and parents to provide advice on positioning and activities, self-help equipment and adaptations to enable the child to attain his optimum level of functioning in his temporary surroundings. It may also be an opportune time to proceed with a period of more intensive therapy than is possible when the child is travelling from home for each treatment session.

The medical social worker will already know the parents of a child whose impairments were apparent at birth. Other parents may have become acquainted with their social worker when their child became acutely ill and was admitted to hospital. Some families have contact with a social worker because of family problems which may have existed before their child was born.

Social workers can help the families who have a child with impairments in two main areas — with practical problems and with personal problems associated with their child. Advice can be given about claiming State benefits due to the parents of children with special needs, such as attendance and mobility allowance. Social workers are also experts on the funds which are available from charitable organisations, both at a national and a local level, which can provide facilities which are not available from the State. Funds may be found, for example, to allow low income families to go on holiday, to provide driving lessons so that a mother may travel independently with her child, or to provide a washing machine or dryer. Social workers will be conversant with the agencies which provide relief care for the families of the severely impaired child which may include facilities which care for the child while the parents and siblings are on holiday, relief when the family is under great stress or simply a babysitter in whom the parents feel sufficient confidence to leave their child while they enjoy an evening out together.

Some parents are well able to cope with the practical aspects of having a child with impairments but welcome the opportunity to discuss with a person who is specially trained the emotional problems which accompany the birth and care of their special child. They can also provide similar help for siblings who can be deeply affected by the birth and the greater amount of attention needed by their sister or brother with impairments.

The occupational therapist should work closely with the social worker so that she is aware of any material, emotional or relationship difficulties which exist within the families she treats. Sometimes the occupational therapist may become aware of problems though they have not been explicitly voiced by parents. She may notice that the parents are particularly tired or stressed. These and many other problems which become apparent during treatment sessions are ones with which the social workers and the occupational therapist may work together to solve.

The educational psychologist will assess and advise on the special educational needs of children with impairments. A school for normal children in the area may supply these needs or it may be necessary, at some stage during the child's years of formal education, to send him to an establishment which has special facilities.

An assessment will be made of his intellectual level as well as other skills which are necessary to function at school such as the length of his concentration span, his distractibility and his self-motivation.

When a child is multiply impaired it is not possible to assess his intellectual abilities and social behaviour in isolation. Decisions regarding his formal education must be taken jointly by his parents and all the professionals who treat him. It is important that the occupational therapist liaises with the educational psychologist so that the child may be approached and asked to respond in a manner which allows him to demonstrate his skills and abilities to the best effect.

There are many other specialists who become involved with the child who has continuing impairment. Some will require the skills of other medical specialists, neurologists, orthopaedic surgeons, urologists, cardiologists, psychiatrists, etc. Other agencies in the community will help the child and his family. Whoever becomes involved must work as part of a team as it is uneconomical of finance, resources and expertise for a team member to work in isolation.

2

A Model for the Process of Learning

> Nature without learning is blind, learning apart from nature is fractional, and practice in the absence of both is aimless
>
> *Plutarch, AD 100*

Infants of four to five months will regard an object which they are manipulating. 'This is the real beginning of all the experimentation and observation which children carry out to find what the world, and the objects in it, are like' (Vernon, 1971, p. 20). Children are, of course, learning from a much earlier age, at least from the moment of birth. The point in the maturational process when a child begins to examine visually an object which he is manipulating must surely be a momentous occasion. The world stimulates curiosity; it becomes reasonable and logical because objects may be classified according to their sensory qualities of appearance, behaviour and use.

The infant is learning probably at a greater rate than he ever will during the remainder of his life. His behaviour is changing rapidly as he understands more of his environment and the objects and people within it. The observation that his behaviour is changing is evidence that he is learning, since 'Learning is the process by which experience changes behaviour. We use the word 'learning', only when the change in behaviour is long-lasting or permanent' (Nathan, 1969, p. 309).

Learning is 'the apparent modification of a person's behaviour through his activities and experiences, so that his knowledge, skills and attitudes, including modes of adjustment, towards his environment are changed, more or less permanently' (Curzon, 1980, p. 7).

LEARNING — THE RESPONSE TO STIMULI

Stimuli may come from the environment — sights, sounds, smells, tastes, tactile sensations — or from within a person, for example when proprioceptive stimuli make a person aware of the position of his limbs without visual reference. Behaviour is the response to such stimuli which may be muscular (movement), involuntary (the response of the automatic nervous system such as the dilation of the pupils) or the response may be purely mental in which case it will be difficult to observe.

Learning does not necessarily take place in formal situations such as school, nursery or playgroup, therapy sessions or dedicated parent/child instruction sessions. It takes place whenever a child is in a state where he is responsive to stimuli from his environment. A child who is able to crawl will sense the coldness of the vinyl when he moves from the carpeted hall to the hard floor of the kitchen. He will learn that he is able to move more quickly on the hard, smooth vinyl which produces less friction than the hall carpet. The child has not been taught the qualities of carpet and vinyl flooring, heat and cold or the effects of friction on movement; but through sensory stimuli he appreciates the relative qualities of hard and soft floors. He adapts his behaviour, in this case movements, appropriately. Through his own efforts he has received stimuli, perceived them and responded by motor activity. He has adapted his behaviour to suit his environment; he has learned.

Therefore, if learning takes place through response to stimuli, a child who has an impairment to the reception of one or more modes of stimulus, imperfect perception or processing of those stimuli or motor incapacity, he will be disadvantaged in both spontaneous and formal learning situations. *The basis of the work of the occupational therapist is, therefore, to enable the child to make the best use of his capacities for learning and to explain and demonstrate to others involved with the child how this may best be achieved.*

In order for the occupational therapist to help children who have disabilities she must understand the nature of the impairment. This understanding may be reached by observing the child during various activities and in situations which are appropriate to his and his family's lifestyle and his maturational level, by listening to his parents account of his behaviour and by the use of standardised tests, the results of which may be compared with the levels attained by children of comparable maturational ages. From this careful observation she will be able to deduce the nature of his disability and the measures which may be taken to increase his abilities. It is not sufficient to observe that a child is unable to perform an activity. The *reasons* for his inability, if not immediately apparent, must be sought and evaluated so that he may be helped to attain his maximum performance level in the whole range of life skills.

DEFINING THE CAUSES OF NON-RESPONSE

There are many reasons for a child's lack of success with activities, the pertinent one not always being the most obvious. A child, for example, may suffer from hemiparesis and have difficulty in performing two-handed activities but perceptual difficulties relating to spatial concepts may prove more significant than his obvious motor impairment. It is important therefore to consider all the possible reasons for lack of success. The following example provides numerous reasons why a child may fail to draw a circle which most three year olds are able to do. Some of the reasons are more probable than others, a few of them are extremely unlikely. The example illustrates the breadth of questioning necessary to define the precise nature of disability. It also shows the importance of the occupational therapist's involvement with other specialists who are experts in specific aspects of child development and disability.

A child is provided with paper and pencil and is asked to draw a circle. Consider the reasons why he may not comply with this request:

1. The child is not attending to the request because he is curious about other objects in the room.
2. He is distracted by noises within or outside the room.
3. He is distracted by the movements of other people or objects.
4. He has impaired hearing and cannot hear the request.
5. He has a visual impairment and has never seen a circle clearly. He cannot see the paper because there is poor definition between its colour and the table on which it has been placed. He cannot locate the pencil for similar reasons. His visual fields are impaired and the pencil is not in a position where he can see it. He only has peripheral vision and cannot see the paper clearly in the middle of the table.
6. He has a receptive language impairment and cannot understand the request.
7. He has perceptual difficulties and does not understand circularity.
8. He has not reached the maturational age (three years) when he is able to draw a circle.

9. He has problems with motor organisation and although he understands the request and the qualities of a circle he is unable to plan his hand movements in order to draw a circle.
10. He cannot pick up the pencil because he cannot bring his arm, and thus his hand, into midline in front of himself.
11. He has flexor spasm and cannot extend his arm to reach for the pencil.
12. Impaired hand function prevents him from picking up the pencil.
13. He is unable to sustain his grip on the pencil.
14. Intention tremor, ataxia or athetosis prevent him from drawing a circle.
15. The child has insufficient muscle power to hold or move the pencil.
16. He has tried previously to draw a circle, failed to do so and is reluctant to try again.
17. His sitting position is unstable, he is afraid of falling and prefers to use his hands to support himself rather than to draw.
18. A timid nervous child may be reluctant to take part in any activities particularly if he is in strange surroundings.
19. If the situation is one of formal assessment the child may feel the tension of his parent's anxiety for him to give his best and feel unable to co-operate.

Some of the above reasons for a child not complying with a request to draw a circle are so obvious that they are unlikely to be considered. An occupational therapist would know immediately if a child was suffering from severe cerebral palsy or if the child had a severe loss of muscle power. It may not be immediately obvious that a child has an impairment of receptive language or problems with motor organisation in the supposedly 'good' hand in instances of hemiparesis. Some children may fail because of a single problem, others may have a combination of difficulties. The *reason* for a child's failure is more important than the fact that he has failed.

The reason for failure in one task will be relevant to other activities. A child who has difficulty aligning pieces of a formboard so that they will fit into the related insets may also have difficulty aligning a button with a buttonhole. A child who needs to monitor visually his hand movements, for example, when he apposes each finger in turn to his thumb, may have difficulty cutting out pictures as this involves the manipulation of the scissors in one hand and the holding and moving of the paper with the other. The child will be unable to monitor visually the movement of both hands simultaneously.

The reasons for a child's failure in specific tasks hold the clues to how he may best be taught and how he will learn in both formal and informal situations. By analysing a child's performance, his successes and failures, the occupational therapist will be able to plan appropriate learning situations for therapy sessions, and at home and at school. She will be able to suggest appropriate self-help equipment, adaptations and strategies so that the child may exploit his abilities during play, self-care, the activities of daily living and in school. She will be able to discuss the child's needs with his parents taking into account their lifestyle and family philosophies, and with his teachers bearing in mind the teaching methods used in that school.

Firstly, the occupational therapist must make decisions regarding the needs of the child. Childhood is a time of rapid growth, not only physical but also rapid increase in skills and abilities, knowledge and experience, relationships and methods of communications. Any impairment of sensory, intellectual or motor function may prevent or impoverish one or more of these aspects of childhood. The occupational therapist should consider the whole life experience of the child when assessing and setting goals which will ultimately modify his learned behaviour so that he may adapt to his environment. One way of achieving this is to consider the complete learning process, beginning with the transmitter of information following the process through to the response to the stimulus.

THE LEARNING PROCESS

The model is partly an educational one and partly one used by many therapists. The educational model is based on a transmitter of stimuli or information and a receiver, the child. As with many methods of communication, there may be 'interference' along the channel between transmitter and receiver. This interference or 'noise', as it is sometimes called, may prevent the reception of the message. Teachers should therefore consider their teaching techniques and their language register (language at an appropriate level of complexity for the receiver). They should look at the physical qualities of the teaching environment, the temperature, humidity, lighting. seating, which, if uncomfortable, could create barriers to learning. They should consider the appropriateness of the material being taught to their pupils' age, experience, level of knowledge and skills and their motivation to learn.

Figure 2.1: The transmission of information to the child

Transmitter →	Interference →	Receiver
(teacher peers, family therapist environment objects)	(barriers to learning)	(child)

This model (see Figure 2.1) is usually applied by teachers to the process of learning in the classroom. It can equally well be applied to any other learning situation. Most young children enjoy playing with water containers in the bath, pouring from one to the other. By repetition of this game the child learns about the qualities of water. The process of pouring has transmitted the message about these qualities and the child has received the message. Perhaps one day the bath water is a little warmer than usual and the child is concentrating on keeping the uncomfortable water as still as possible. On that occasion the heat of the bath water will be a barrier to learning.

The model is also an appropriate one to apply to children who have one or more impairments. With such children consideration must be given to the manner in which messages are transmitted:

1. Is the information such that it may be received by the child?
2. Is it in a mode which may be received by the unimpaired sensory channels of the child?
3. Complex verbal information will not be received by a child who has difficulty with the comprehension of the spoken word.
4. Some transmitted visual information will not be received by a child who has a visual field defect.

Children who have impairments may have more barriers to learning than the average child. They may be prevented from receiving information by the interference they themselves create. The movement and noise of athetosis or the inability to maintain a stable sitting position could become barriers to learning.

When we talk of a child as a receiver of information we also imply the part of a child concerned with sensory input. The problems of the child with continuing disability should be considered in the logical sequence of sensory input, gnosis, perception and other intellectual activity, praxis and motor response (see Figure 2.2)

Figure 2.2: Processing information

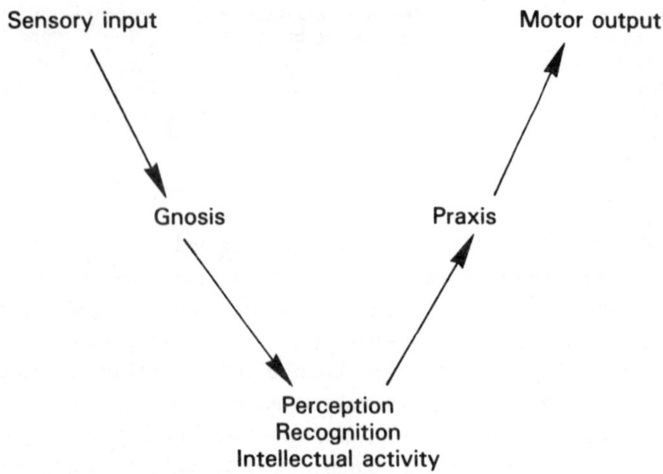

By analysing a child's response to stimuli or information, by presenting material in different modes and by discussing the child with other specialists it will be possible for the occupational therapist to find the break or breaks in the chain between sensory input and motor output. She will then be able to plan her therapy, self-help equipment and adaptations to the best effect for a particular child.

Combining these two models provides a basis on which the child's abilities and problems may be analysed and strategies formed to enable him to gain the maximum amount of information from his environment and to respond to that information appropriately (see Figure 2.3).

The model may be applied to formal learning situations, learning the skills of daily living, play activity or at any time when the child is in an alert receptive and responsive state. It is useful for devising the best methods for a particular child of learning a complex activity such as feeding or for a single element of an activity such as maintaining the head in mid-line.

The model is self-perpetuating because the successful transmission of messages, their assimilation and appropriate response to them, elicits the transmission of further messages and responses. Thus the child is communicating and such responses lead to learning when his behaviour is changed, more or less permanently.

Figure 2.3: The learning model as applied to the child with impairments

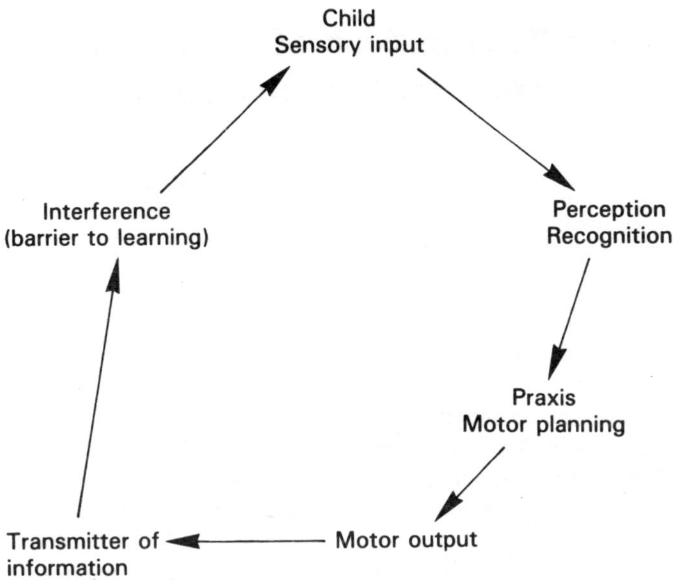

3

The Transmission of Information Appropriate to the Child

There is a poignancy in all things clear,
In the stare of the deer, in the ring of a
hammer in the morning.
Seeing a bucket of perfectly lucid water
We fall to imagining prodigious honesties.

Richard Wilbur "Clearness", Ceremony (1950)

An eight-year-old boy who had severe learning difficulties was struggling with a reading test. None of his attempts were successful. The test administrator preparing to conclude the test tried to give him clues to the last word which was 'school', so that he could end on a note of success. 'This is a word you see outside a place you go to with your mummy nearly every day. It is written on a board in big letters.' The boy looked puzzled for a moment then his face lit up with a flash of inspiration. 'I know, I know what it says. It says pub!'

Now obviously the test administrator had not transmitted appropriate information for this boy, it was ambiguous. How had the boy arrived at his answer? Perhaps his parents had verbalised the idea to him. Perhaps the idea was transmitted to him by overhearing snatches of his parents conversation. Maybe he had often accompanied his parents to a public house and perceived it as the place the family visited most often. He may have frequently smelled alcohol on his parents breath. There are numerous ways in which this boy may have come to his answer. He may have heard about it, seen it, smelled the results of the visit. In some way the information was transmitted to him and led him to deduce that this was the place the reading test administrator had in mind.

This tale illustrates some of the many ways in which information is transmitted to children. It illustrates some of the ways in which learning takes place. Transmitters of information are not only people but also objects and the environment — sounds, movements, tastes and smells.

Information is not only transmitted in formal situations, in school, by parents and therapy sessions. Information is continually being transmitted from a variety of sources, its effectiveness will depend on whether it is appropriate for the receiver, which is especially important for the child who has one or more disabilities. For such a child it may be necessary to adapt the transmission of information so that he may assimilate it. Adaptation may be necessary to: the child's environment; his toys and equipment; the level and mode of language which is used to address him.

THE ENVIRONMENT

A child who has a disability may not be free to gain the maximum amount of information from his environment, it may be necessary to adapt it to his needs. The occupational therapist must ensure that the environment during her therapy sessions is suitable for the child.

1. The child who is easily distracted.
   (a) It may be necessary to exclude people other than the child and herself from the treatment room.
   (b) There should be no noise outside the room which could distract the child.
   (c) It may be necessary to draw curtains or lower blinds and rely on artificial light in order to eliminate visual distraction.
   (d) The room should be clear of toys and equipment which may distract the child.
   (e) The test piece of equipment or toy should be presented alone, the rest being kept out of view of the child until required.
2. The child who is difficult to stimulate.
   (a) The presence of parents or siblings who can work with the therapist to relate activities to familiar situations can provide valuable stimulation.
   (b) It does not follow that a 'busy' environment will stimulate the child who lacks motivation and interest. Such a child will respond more readily to a stimulus directed to his most responsive sensory channel. For example, the child who responds to sound may be

drawn into the desired activity by a musical toy whose possibilities include the use of other skills such as leading with the index finger, or pronation and supination of wrist.

Case note

Sarah suffered a severe convulsion at the age of two and a half years following which she was put on anti-convulsive therapy. There followed several more severe convulsions and subsequent adjustments in her drug regime.

Sarah was referred for occupational therapy because of slow progress in school, lethargy and a severe tremor which affected her ability to use a pencil. A weighted bracelet was used effectively to reduce her tremor and a triangular pencil grip was introduced to encourage a tripod pencil grip. Although Sarah always co-operated to the best of her ability she had a low level of motivation and lacked self-confidence. Both motivation and self-confidence improved dramatically when her older brother and her special friend from school were included in therapy sessions. Although these two boys were employed with their own drawings, their presence stimulated Sarah to attempt new tasks. The display of their drawings on the walls of the therapy room stimulated her to try new ideas and effects in her drawings.

The occupational therapist will suggest ways in which the home or some part of it may be modified or augmented to provide the best form of stimulation for the child.

Sensory deficit

The most common sensory deficits are those of vision and hearing, many of which are difficult to diagnose and define precisely in the multiply impaired child. Occupational therapists should always familiarise themselves with the findings of other professionals who work with a child and take into account their findings. They should also be alert to the possibility of undiagnosed visual and auditory deficits.

Case note

Ruth is seven years old and suffers from athetoid cerebral palsy and a moderately severe high frequency hearing loss. She is of normal intelligence and highly motivated to succeed. Her poor hand function leads to great frustration particularly when attempting to draw and paint. In order to allow her to produce some artwork which would satisfy her own high standards, her occupational therapist encouraged her to use simple printing techniques using potato cuts and commercially available rubber stamps of geometric shapes and outlines of animals, flowers, fruit, etc. On one occasion her therapist had drawn the trunk and branches of a tree, intending Ruth to print the leaves. She obviously did not understand what was required of her. Initially her therapist wondered if the difficulty was being caused by her hearing loss and not understanding instructions. It was found that the real problem was because of an undiagnosed visual problem. Ruth had extra-pyramidal signs and gazing upwards caused her discomfort, hence she had only seen trees from a distance and had not appreciated their individual leaves. Subsequently it was discovered that she had only seen television aerials attached to chimneys in the distance because of this visual problem. In the school situation her occupational therapist was able to point out to her teacher the difficulty she would experience if she were required to look up to a chalkboard or other types of visual display, particularly if she was sitting near to them.

Visual factors

Poor visual acuity and defects of the visual field will limit the child's view of his environment.

1. It may be necessary to draw a child's attention to certain items or to move him into positions where he may see them.
2. Objects may be more clearly seen against a strongly contrasting background.
3. Some colours may be more easily seen than others. The occupational therapist will need to experiment with each child to discover which colours are most easily seen by him. Frequently red or yellow will be found to be good choices. Some children respond well to highly reflective metallic finishes.
4. The child may require a high degree of illumination to be able to fully appreciate his environment or he may respond well to highly reflective materials.
5. Other children may be more responsive when working in a darkened room with only the parts of the room or objects being used illuminated.

Sound

Children also learn a great deal from the sounds of their environment. When the sound of cooking equipment is heard food is likely to be forthcoming. When the sound of a car is heard in the drive followed by the noise of the garage door opening, the child knows his father will soon appear in the house. Most children look expectantly when they hear a sweet paper crackle. Some children who have an impairment of hearing may need to have their attention drawn to such sequences of events. Others may have problems concentrating on one source of sound in an environment where there are a number of sounds — figure background difficulty. For such children care should be taken to exclude extraneous sounds from the therapy room.

Touch

Children learn about their environment by touching but a child who, because of a disability, is unable to touch, handle and manipulate, is deprived of a great deal of spontaneous learning. A child whose hand is fisted by spasticity or whose arm is held in flexion and can only be reduced by conscious effort will be deprived of much tactile stimulation. The child who is unable to move himself freely within his environment will miss much of the touching usually experienced in childhood.

Of course, tactile experience is not restricted to the hands. Although the hands, and particularly the finger tips, contain especially sensitive tactile receptors, the whole of the body is sensitive to tactile stimulation. This point is particularly pertinent to any child who is unable to move freely within his environment. The child who suffers cerebral palsy may not be ambulant and may need help with every change of position. His parents will take care that he is comfortable, neither too hot or too cold, that he is protected from the elements and all conceivable dangers. No parent could be criticised for such diligent care of a child. However, the child will probably never experience much of the tactile stimulation which is available to other children. When he is taken outside he may be so well protected that he has never felt the rain, snow or wind on his face. He may never have put his feet on grass or felt the hardness of a stone beneath them. He will never have been scolded for playing with mud so he is also unlikely to appreciate its tactile properties. He may be able to see that leaves turn from green to yellow and brown in the autumn but he may not appreciate that they change from being sappy and pliable to being dry and brittle.

Often it is not possible for the severely disabled child to share every experience with his able-bodied peers. It is important that those concerned with the child are aware of the normal range of tactile experiences and facilitate a wide range of experience for him. The occupational therapist who is especially concerned with activities of daily living is in an ideal position to encourage such experience and to discuss with the child's parents how they, in their ordinary day to day activities, may also increase their child's experience of his environment.

TOYS AND EQUIPMENT

Children learn through play. They learn about the quality of materials, about construction, about a variety of concepts which will later be integrated into everyday life. Children use imagination whilst playing and work out interpersonal relationships. During play activities children develop their skills of observation and concentration, motor, sensory and perceptual skills. The child who has one or more disabilities may not be free to play.

The occupational therapist will be able to suggest suitable toys for such children, adapt commercially available ones or design a toy which will have a specific purpose for a child. She may collaborate with other therapists who are involved with the child in adapting or designing toys which will serve a number of purposes.

In other instances the occupational therapist may work together with technicians to produce a toy which can become a transmitter of information for a child. Today it is possible, by the use of electronic techniques, to compensate for a child's motor deficit so that he may control toys. The use of touch pads and custom designed switches which may be operated by hand, foot, head and almost any other part of the body, have extended the experiences of many children who have disabilities (Heddell, 1985, pp. 25–38),

The nature of the play material will, of course, be considered in the light of the child's disabilities. Points which have already been mentioned when discussing the child's environment will require consideration:

1. Toys must be appropriate to a child's intellectual and developmental levels.
2. They should be selected bearing in mind his visual acuity. Their

position must be carefully chosen if the child has a visual field defect.
3. The toy must be sufficiently interesting to attract and maintain the child's attention.
4. The effort of controlling or manipulating the toy should not detract from the motivation to continue the activity.

Qualities of play materials which may affect the child's ability to learn from them

1. The weight of toys relative to a child's condition is important. The child who has muscle weakness associated with conditions such as the spinal muscular atrophies and congenital myopathies need lightweight toys. Conversely, the child who is ataxic or has a tremor may manipulate toys more effectively if their weight and thus gravity is increased. It may be necessary to reach the optimum weight increase by trial and error.
2. The child who has only a limited range of movement in his arms will need compact toys which can be used in a small space. Those with delay in the development of manipulation will often cope best with scaled up versions of toys.
3. Children with severe developmental delay will need toys to suit their developmental level but of a size to suit their physical stature. This will entail making large versions of toys usually used by much younger children.
4. Children are interested in the textures of various materials and it is important that all children are given a wide range of tactile experiences. Children who have difficulty with manipulation may find some textures easier to handle than others. A degree of friction on the surface of a toy, such as felt rather than shiny plastic, may enable a child to grasp it more securely. For the same reason a matt finish on a wooden toy is often preferable to a glossy varnished or painted one.
5. The controls of mechanical and electronic toys will require adapting to suit the needs of the child. Knobs and handles may need to be enlarged or their shape altered to suit the most effective grip of a particular child. The direction in which knobs and handles need to be turned, pushed, or pulled may need adjusting so that they use the child's most effective and desirable pattern of movement.

Case note

Richard suffers from ataxic cerebral palsy. He had been tre the occupational, speech and physiotherapists on a twice w basis until he began attending school at the age of five years. occupational therapist had adapted a number of toys for him increasing their weight so that he could handle them more easily. She had also devised a number of matching games where he could point to the appropriate object or picture card so that his perceptual skills could be assessed and where necessary practice in them provided. Before he entered school he was able to match colours and select named ones, understand more than and less than, demonstrate his understanding of prepositions, numbers up to five, size, shape, position in space and spacial relationships.

Before he began school his teachers were invited to the clinic to observe his abilities and discuss his special needs with his therapists. When he had been in school for a few weeks, his occupational therapist visited him to observe how he was faring in the classroom rather than a one-to-one situation, and to discuss any difficulties with his teacher.

Richard was working on number concept, matching the spots on number cards with the appropriate number of small plastic toys. He was not meeting with great success which his teacher had interpreted as inability to match numbers. In fact his problems arose because the number cards he had been given were too small and the toys he had been given were inappropriate for his manipulative skills. When his small number cards were replaced by A4 sized ones with spots 5 cm in diameter and the small hollow plastic toys were replaced by small but comparatively heavy metal cars he was able to demonstrate his ability to match numbers. When the transmitters of information, the materials which Richard was to work with, were appropriate to his needs he was able to demonstrate his potential.

THE MODE AND LEVEL OF LANGUAGE

Any form of language is a system of symbols by which information is passed between people. There must be a transmitter of those symbols and a receiver who is able to decode them. The symbols of language may be spoken or written words. There are several basic principles which should be considered when transmitting information to the child with sensory impairment.

The position of the child and the therapist

1. Ensure that the communicator is on the same level as the child. An adult will need to kneel or sit on the floor when speaking to a small child who is standing. If the child is sitting at a table, a chair a little lower than the child's will bring both to a similar level.
2. It is usually best for an adult to be positioned directly opposite the child, for thus it is possible to attain and maintain physical contact and for toys and equipment to be presented in the child's mid-line. It also ensures that the child may see the communicator without altering his sitting position — an important consideration for the child who needs to be placed and supported in order to be able to attend to and manipulate equipment. A person addressing such a child from his left or right would cause the child to attempt to turn to that side, often unbalancing his sitting position which he cannot right himself.
3. For the child who has auditory or visual deficits it is important that the person addressing him sits with their face in a good light. A child with a degree of deafness will probably watch a speaker's face and lip movements more closely than a child with perfect hearing. The occupational therapist concerned with the child must consult with whoever has assessed his hearing so that she understands the degree of deafness from which he suffers and the frequencies at which he hears best. A child with a high frequency loss may hear more of what is said to him if the pitch of the voice is lowered slightly. He may have difficulty hearing particular consonant sounds such as *s*, *p*, *b*. When it is necessary to use words beginning with such sounds, knowledge of the child's problem enables the therapist to say the words particularly clearly, choose alternative words or back up the words with gesture or demonstration.
4. A child with visual problems will also need good lighting in order to see as clearly as possible the person who is addressing him and to be able to see any equipment which is being shown to him. Some visually handicapped children are encouraged to concentrate on what is being said to them if the speaker wears something made from highly reflective material which maintains their visual attention. Sitting or kneeling opposite a child also helps to concentrate his attention to what is being said to him. There are children who have little difficulty understanding what is being said to them but have problems concentrating on the spoken word. Other children can only understand the spoken word when they are giving their full attention. Concentration is more likely to be maintained if the speaker is

opposite and has good eye contact with the child.
5. There are occasions when it would be easier for the communicator to sit alongside the child, for example when both are engaged in writing or drawing. It takes little time and effort to learn to write and draw upside down, and it is a skill well worth practising in order to keep a face to face position with the child.

The level of language used to address the child

The level and complexity of the verbal language used to address the child should also be considered. The occupational therapist should understand and ideally discuss the findings of the speech therapist so that she may address the child at an appropriate level. She should note if his understanding of spoken language is delayed, if it is similar to a younger child, or if it is deviant, i.e. experiencing difficulties not normally encountered in the development of language comprehension. He may have difficulty understanding a sentence with a number of elements and require it to be broken down into its components, each presented separately. He may have difficulty sequencing the words in a sentence though he understands the individual words. Mis-sequencing of a sentence completely alters its meaning. Some children have difficulty with prepositions such as, in, on, beside, under, etc. Occupational therapists treating a child's perceptual difficulties would be particularly interested in discussing such comprehension difficulties with the speech therapist so that together they could decide if the problem is purely one of language, being able to understand the verbal label for these prepositions, or if it also involves the perceptual concepts.

Language and formal test instructions

Formal tests which the occupational therapist may administer could be invalidated if the child does not understand test instructions. The occupational therapist's test of visual perception could be misinterpreted and the child diagnosed as having perceptual difficulties when in fact he has difficulties with the comprehension of language. Standardised tests are not valid if words other than those in the test instructions are used. If a child has problems with the understanding of language it may become necessary to augment verbal instructions with additional words or demonstrations. The results thus obtained will be useful in assessing the child's abilities but they will not provide the standardised results calculated by the author of the test.

It is not only in the administration of standardised tests that knowledge of the child's level of understanding of the spoken word is important. All occupational therapy administered with the knowledge of the child's level of language comprehension will be more effective. Not only will she help the child and make the most of his abilities but she will also provide an excellent model for parents of how they too may effectively address their child.

Non-verbal communication

Some children are not able to receive normal verbally transmitted information. One group of such children is the profoundly deaf. The occupational therapist should familiarise herself with the plans which have been made about the method or methods of communication which the child will use so that her contact with him will reinforce the work of the agencies.

In recent years children with other types of disabilities have benefitted from being taught non-verbal methods of communication. Sign systems are being used to augment the verbal language of children who have specific difficulties with comprehension and/or expressive language difficulties. It has been found that if these children are provided with an alternative means of communication the imperativeness is removed from verbal language and as a result there is often a spontaneous improvement in it.

Sign systems, particularly Makaton, have been used very successfully with children who are mentally handicapped. It has been found to improve both their comprehension and execution of language. Although some of the children who now use signing to augment their language skills have no difficulty with the comprehension of verbal language. It has been found that it is profitable for those speaking to them to sign simultaneously so that the child's sign vocabulary is reinforced and increased.

There are also children unable to communicate verbally whose poor hand function prevents them from making signs. These children are often taught to use communication boards on which are inscribed pictures, symbols or words which are arranged so that the child may point to phrases or sentences in order to communicate. Again the occupational therapist should be familiar with these systems so that she may speak and simultaneously point to the appropriate word sign or symbol.

Some of the systems of non-verbal communication are as follows:

Sign systems

Makaton is a system of hand signs which is based on British signs. The vocabulary follows a developmental language programme. It is widely used with children who are mentally handicapped (Walker, 1985).

Paget-Gorman is a sign system which follows the rules of English grammar. Its users require good manual dexterity. It has proved to be useful for children with aphasia and other allied disorders.

Amerind is based on the 'hand talk' of the American Indians. Signs are based on concepts rather than individual words or grammatical constructions.

Cued speech is used in conjunction with oral speech. It enables the deaf child to overcome some of the ambiguities of lip reading.

Graphic systems

Blissymbolics may be displayed on a simple board or used in conjunction with an electronic communication aid. The system uses symbols to denote the various parts of speech. It is grammatical although it is not possible to denote many of the subtleties of grammatical construction; for instance, there is only one past tense. It requires more symbolic understanding than pictures or photographs but less than is needed to appreciate the written word.

Pictures and/or the written word are used to form communication systems for the non-verbal child. The simplest are clear photographs which represent objects and actions. For the child who is able to read, words may also be used in the form of a chart or written as required on a typewriter, electronic printer or a VDU.

FACTORS WHICH MAY IMPEDE THE RECEPTION OF STIMULI

Atmospheric interference causes noise which impedes the listeners ability to hear a radio transmission. The signal transmitted may be perfect, as may be the listener's hearing, yet the noise between output and input prevents perfect reception. This analogy may be applied to any learning situation, formal or informal. The 'noise' is not necessarily auditory, it is any mode of interference which intervenes between the transmitter of a stimulus or information and the receiver of it.

The receiver of the stimulus or information must be one or more of the sensory input channels. These receptors are also sensitive to other stimuli which may have a greater impact than the intended one. A child in a classroom may be diverted from the intended task by the temperature of the room, by uncomfortable humidity, poor illumination or dazzling sunlight. The classroom may be overcrowded and the child disturbed by the proximity of his neighbours. The classroom may be badly arranged so that some children have difficulty seeing relevant materials or the teacher.

Many of these constraints may also apply to less formal situations in the home or during outdoor play. Additional factors may include the child's physical and mental state. A child who is not 100 per cent fit may not have the energy to explore his environment despite situations which he usually finds exciting, Recent chastisement by a parent may preoccupy a child and reduce his awareness of his environment. Fatigue or hunger may be uppermost in his mind.

These factors may also form a barrier between the transmission of a stimulus and its response in children who have one or more disabilities. They may, in fact, be more sensitive than the average child to these constraints. There may be other barriers to learning which are dependent on the impairments.

Lack of physical security

There are many disabling conditions of childhood which inflict an extra load on learning. Neurological abnormalities prevent children holding their heads in mid-line, bringing their hands together in midline or maintaining trunk balance. These, and many other skills, need to be learned. Some children will never become proficient in maintaining their posture and will require aids to help them.

Inability to perform two tasks simultaneously

Abnormal postures and patterns of movement require treatment which will require the child's total concentration. He will, for example, not be able to practise sitting balance *and* perform a task requiring him to match objects. Many children who suffer from cerebral palsy are unable to walk and talk at the same time, each task requiring their complete concentration.

Case note

Despite suffering from moderately severe spastic cerebral palsy, Amy was ambulant with the aid of orthoses when she started occupational therapy at the age of five years. Her IQ was within the average range. Walking required her full concentration so she was unable to walk and talk simultaneously.

She was a fashion-conscious little girl and both she and her mother were concerned about her excessive drooling which caused her dresses to become uncomfortably wet, unsightly and at times smelly. A programme was initiated to encourage lip closure and regular swallowing of saliva with the help of a battery operated 'bleep' which reminded her to swallow every 30 seconds. It was hoped that eventually she would become conditioned to swallowing regularly thus removing the excess saliva from her mouth. The programme was effective while Amy was involved in activities which required only a low level of concentration; it failed when she was introduced to an electric typewriter which required complete concentration. She was unable to participate in the two activities simultaneously.

Amy is now twelve years old and with maturation and self-motivation she has overcome her drooling problem in all but the most stressful situations.

In other conditions such as muscular dystrophy and spinal muscular atrophy weak trunk muscles will require support if the child is to be free to observe, play and learn.

Inability to adjust position or to make discomfort known

Consider how frequently an able person adjusts his or her sitting position. A child who needs to be supported in order to maintain an upright posture is not able to make these constant adjustments. He may not be able, because of communication difficulties, to make his discomfort known. Such discomfort, perhaps caused by sitting for a prolonged period on creased clothing, can occupy a child's full attention and form a very real but unobservable barrier to learning.

Consider also the number of different sitting postures which the average person adopts in the course of a day — sometimes erect and sometimes flexed forward over a work surface. Most people spend some time relaxing even semi-reclining in a soft upholstered chair. A child who is not able to adjust his position freely may spend a considerable amount of time in the same chair which, because of the support required, is not constructed from yielding materials. The constant contact with hard materials may make the child very much aware of his own body and its contact with the hard surfaces so that he is distracted from other stimuli.

The child's own involuntary movements

There are many conditions in which one symptom is involuntary movement.

Athetosis

Athetosis can become a barrier between the transmission of stimuli and their reception. It is frequently accompanied by high frequency deafness and the extraneous noise caused by athetoid feet in shoes on a hard floor or the metal footrest of a wheelchair may further impair the reception of auditory stimuli. A thick rug or a piece of carpet which is securely fixed beneath the child's table, covering the area where he could place his feet, will help to reduce the noise his involuntary movements make on a hard floor. The foot rests of a wheelchair could also be lined with foam-backed carpet to reduce the noise of his athetoid movements on the metal.

Hyperactivity

Hyperactivity by its nature causes movement which inhibits learning. The correct sizes of tables and chairs can help to reduce the child's rocking and squirming movements. Chairs should be of such height that his feet are supported on the floor in a plantigrade position with his knees at right angles. The chair should be of a suitable depth to support his thighs. A non-slip surface on the seat will inhibit some of his wriggling movements. A horizontal extension to the back legs of the chair will prevent it being tipped backwards.

Relative size of equipment

Having established that the child is seated or otherwise positioned in the best way for him to concentrate on a task and so that he feels secure, it is necessary to consider the height of the child in relation to his working surface. This surface may be a table, a tray attached to his chair or the floor if he is working in a prone position over a wedge. For a profoundly handicapped child the working surface may also provide part of the support which he needs to maintain his position such as a table or a tray with a cutout.

The height of work surfaces will depend upon the task being undertaken. One slightly higher than is usual will help the child with a tremor keep his forearm in a supported position during such activities as cutting out with scissors. The child with athetosis or dystonia may be helped in the same way or it may be found that a lower table is more effective as it enables him to stabilise his arm by bearing weight through it.

The height of the work surfaces will also be affected by the height of equipment and toys in use. The distance between the lap and adducted elbows is very small in young children. The distance filled by the child's lap, the depth of the table, the height of equipment, and the comfortable level of the child's arms when working are crucial. This is especially so for many children suffering from spina bifida who have a very short trunk. Sometimes the problem takes on another dimension if the child is also obese which requires the table to be placed further away from him thus reducing the reach of his arms. In such instances the arrangement of equipment leaves little room for manoeuvre.

Consider, for example, the child with spina bifida who is using a typewriter or computer. Depending on his age and, therefore, his overall size there may be less than 10 cm. between his lap and the optimum height of his hands for using the keyboard. The thickness of the table on which the machine rests is likely to be between 2 and 3 cm, the depth at the front of a computer keyboard will be about 5 cm, and many typewriters are deeper. The child must be very accurately positioned if he is to be able to work comfortably. A few centimetres of error and the child could be attempting to work with his hands at shoulder level and hardly able to see over the keyboard.

These considerations do not apply to computers and typewriters alone. Any piece of equipment must be arranged in the best position for the child. It is often small young children who are offered toys such as posting boxes during assessment and treatment. Many of these are about 12 cm high, which places the lid through which the pieces are to be posted beyond the sight and even the hands of many children. It is of course possible to hold the box for the child at such an angle that he may see the top. How much more practical it would be if some of these boxes were made with the sides of a wedge shape from which the point had been cut. The lid would then be angled towards the child (Figure 3.1)

Figure 3.1: A wedge-shaped posting box, angled towards the child, making it easier for him to see the lid and post the shapes

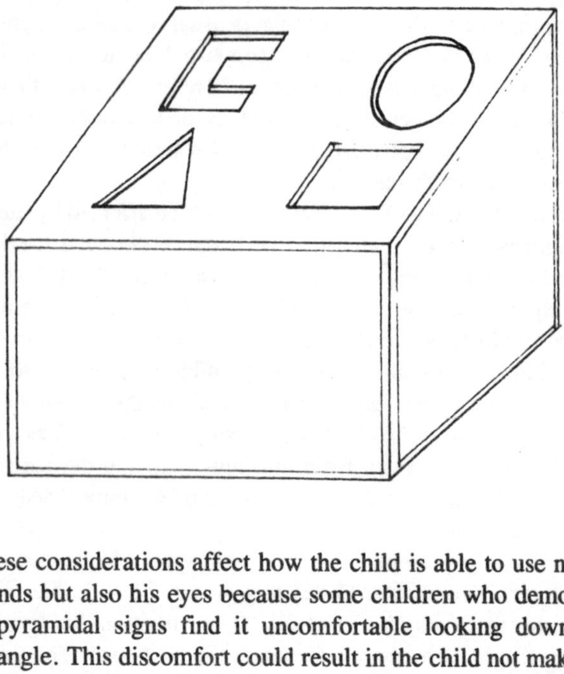

These considerations affect how the child is able to use not only his hands but also his eyes because some children who demonstrate extra-pyramidal signs find it uncomfortable looking down at an acute angle. This discomfort could result in the child not making the best use of information from his environment and equipment.

Case note

Joanna had just completed her first year in secondary school when she suffered a serious road traffic accident. During the next couple of months she made an almost miraculous recovery of her gross motor skills, her comprehension and expression of language. Her fine motor ability was impaired by a gross tremor. As she was already conversant with the QWERTY keyboard, her occupational therapist spent several sessions teaching her the correct fingering.

Using a typewriter with a keyguard she quickly became proficient. She had little difficulty looking slightly down to the platen of the typewriter to read her typing. She continued, however, to have difficulty reading a book which was placed flat on the table in front of her; acute downward gaze was very uncomfortable. She was helped by the provision of a book stand which supported reading material at approximately 60 degrees to the horizontal.

The occupational therapist has very important decisions to make regarding her basic approach to these children. She holds the keys to many areas of learning and she is able to facilitate the removal of many, though not all, barriers. She must study the variety of theories of treatment which are available and use her skill and knowledge to extract the elements which are pertinent to a particular child and his family. She should even consider the effect of no treatment. Would some children find the means to remove their own barriers to learning? (Taft, 1972)

4

The Senses and Sensory Problems

Making terms with reality, with things as they are, is a full-time business for the child.

Milton R. Sapirstein, Paradoxes of Everyday Life (1955)

All that is experienced, all that is learned, everything which results in emotional reactions must first pass through one of the channels of sensory input. Making sense of the environment, moving within it, manipulating equipment, communication between two or more people, requires the use of one or more senses. For most of the time vast numbers of sensory stimuli are received, recognised, acted upon or ignored without conscious effort on the part of the person receiving them.

The child who has unimpaired sensory input, unless he is mentally handicapped, does not need to be taught how to see, hear, taste, smell, appreciate tactile sensations, proprioception, temperature, pain and pressure. With these sensations he is able to learn about himself, his environment and the people within it. Should there be a major impairment of one of the senses in the absence of other impairments, it is likely to be observed by both parents and professionals. A less severe impairment of one of the senses may not be immediately observable and one which is accompanied by other severe impairments may not be immediately sought, particularly if other impairments require prompt treatment such as a lesion of spina bifida which requires immediate surgical closure, or severe feeding problems in a child suffering from cerebral palsy.

The occupational therapist, therefore, should take the diagnosed sensory impairments into account and be alert to the possibility of undiagnosed ones when assessing children's abilities or planning and administering treatment.

VISION

Few children are born with absolutely no vision, though many have severely impaired vision which if not stimulated in the early years will never become useful. Children who have severe visual impairment will not only be unable to use vision as a channel by which information is received but they will also be slower in other areas of development because of their sensory impairment (Dreier, 1980). They will not be stimulated visually to explore their environment nor will they be able to use vision to learn about their own position in space or their relationship to other objects and people.

Such children will need encouragement to explore their own bodies and learn its schema. They will prefer to be in positions where a large percentage of their body is in contact with a hard surface to the extent that their spontaneous means of locomotion may be a supine position arching the back and pushing back on the head. They may, therefore, be delayed in their ability to sit unsupported and to creep. The progression from standing whilst holding a firm object to walking may be especially slow. Many will need help to explore objects by touch, to manipulate them and to reach out to touch and explore surfaces in their environment. Concepts such as the constancy of objects require special attention.

It has been found beneficial to begin treating these children in the first few months of life so that these basic skills may be encouraged and their importance explained to parents as being the basis on which more complex skills of independence will be built. Treatment in group situations is helpful for these children who my be isolated because of their severe impairment. Parents also find these situations beneficial because they meet others whose children are experiencing similar difficulties and they provide mutual support especially during inevitable periods of depression.

Stimulating the child with severe visual impairment

1. Always approach the child gently, talk to him as he is approached. Change his position slowly, talking through the movements. Hold him in such a way that he feels secure. If adults who handle him regularly wear perfume they should always wear the same one so that the child will learn to recognise it.
2. Encourage the child to explore his own body. Tie a ribbon on which a small bell is threaded around his wrist or ankle thus using

an auditory channel to draw his attention to his limbs and to encourage him to bring his two hands together or his hands to his feet.

3. Encourage him to explore his parents' face, hair, hands and body.
4. Study reports of the child's visual abilities and disabilities so that he can be approached and people and toys can be presented in the position and at the distance at which he best sees them.
5. Use toys with a noise element to gain the child's interest and to encourage him to search for them. In the first instance they should be within his reach and, if necessary, his hands should be guided to them until he becomes aware of the space around him and knows that it may contain interesting objects. Later toys may be placed a little further away from the child who should be encouraged to search for them. The noise of the toy will help him to develop skills of locating the direction of a sound.
6. Offer toys with interesting shapes and textures to encourage him to explore them with his hands.
7. Choose toys which will stimulate the child to use any vision he possesses.
   (a) Experiment to discover which colours he can see most easily.
   (b) Choose toys which have fluorescent colours.
   (c) Shine the beam of a torch on toys which have reflective surfaces, such as Christmas tree baubles (see Figure 4.1).
   (d) Cover cubes and other toys which have flat surfaces with refractive paper.
8. Ensure that the background against which a toy is presented is of a strong contrast.
   (a) Plain backgrounds for floors and tables will make the toy easier to see than a patterned one in which the toy may be 'lost'.
   (b) Use backgrounds which are of a strong colour contrast to the toy.
   (c) Some children respond best if the area where they are working is strongly illuminated and the rest of the room is dark.
9. Co-ordination of hand and eye may be encouraged by teaching the child to operate a touch switch or joy stick which controls coloured lights.
10. Disco lights which are illuminated for pre-set times and sequences encourage the child to look in various directions.
11. A computer with a visual display unit and a very simple colour programme will encourage some children to concentrate visually and to co-ordinate hand and eye by operating a control to continue the programme.

Figure 4.1: A torch beam shone on to the reflective surface of a Christmas tree bauble to attract the visual attention of a severely visually handicapped child

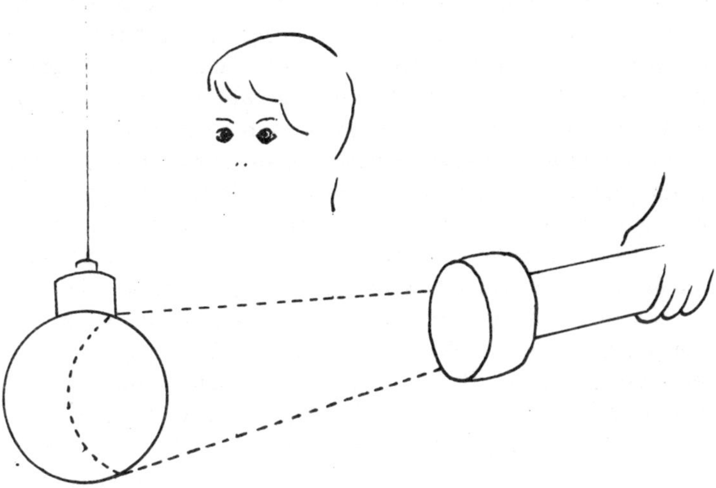

Case note

Within a few weeks of his birth, John's parents noticed that he was not using his eyes as they would have expected and that his general movements seemed 'odd'. Neurological examination suggested that he was probably suffering from ataxia and that he has very little useful vision. He later proved to have a severe articulatory speech problem. From that time he was seen regularly by speech, physiotherapists and occupational therapists and an orthoptist. Because of his severe and diverse problems, it was impossible to make clear predictions at that time about his intellectual level.

Occupational therapy aimed to:

1. Increase his attention span.
2. Encourage eye-hand co-ordination.
3. Provide toys appropriate to his developmental level which he was able to see and handle despite his ataxia.
4. Develop his perceptual skills.
5. Discuss with his parents how best to help him by providing a suitable environment, by the way they handled him and by the provision of suitable toys.

By the age of three years it was apparent that his vision was improving, no doubt due in part to the stimulation he had received. He was able to walk with an unsteady broad-based gait. John continued to be a difficult child to work with because he was so easily frustrated by his inabilities, particularly his poor hand skills and the difficulty he had making himself understood verbally. He was very much aware of the areas where he had difficulty and refused to attempt tasks at which he feared failure. In retrospect it can be seen that his 'difficult' behaviour was an indication of his intellectual skills which at that time were not manifest.

John is now eight years old and attends a unit within a normal primary school for children with language difficulties. He has made normal progress with reading. He uses an electric typewriter with normal-sized print to record his school work because his poor fine motor skills preclude handwriting. The other children in his class have a notebook in which their teacher writes the spellings of unfamiliar words. John has difficulty turning flimsy paper pages so his spellings are recorded in an alphabetical telephone number book which springs open at the required page when the appropriate lettered button is pressed. (see Figure 4.2). His occupational therapist visits his school periodically to monitor his typing skills and to suggest solutions to any minor problems which arise as new skills are required for academic progression.

His ataxia continues to cause problems during Physical Education classes and with dressing. Intellectually he has now been assessed as bright average. The hours of stimulation which he received during his early years from his parents and therapists has, in the long term, proved to have been highly effective, particularly the stimulation of his vision which for the first two years of his life seemed to be minimal.

Occupational therapists have an important role to play in early stimulation and the encouragement of progression through the stages of sensory, motor and perceptual development of the child with visual impairment. 'Occupational therapy deals . . . with complete play- or handling-patterns which are necessary for the child to cope with daily-life practical situations' (Dreier, 1980). Many of the motor activities of the normal infant must be taught to the child with severe visual impairment. They require prolonged encouragement and special strategies to move to explore their environment and to develop useful grasp with which to examine and learn about the nature of objects. Perceptual-cognitive skills require prolonged

Figure 4.2: A telephone book with press button opening may be used as a spelling file for children who have difficulty turning the flimsy pages of a note book

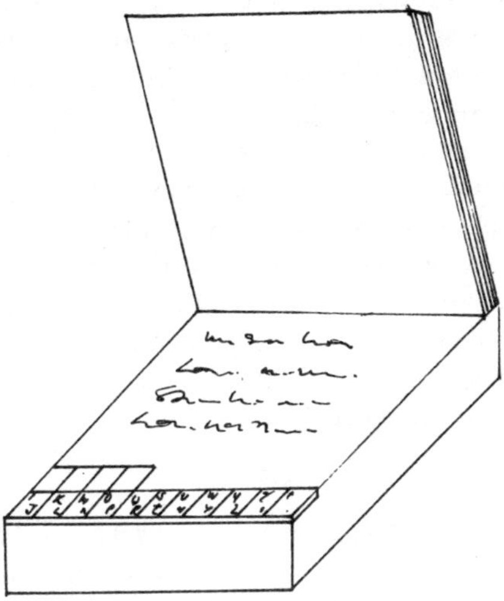

patient encouragement so that more than one sense may be used at the same time. At a later stage the occupational therapist will be concerned with the child's increasing independence in the areas of feeding, dressing and other personal skills.

The majority of children who occupational therapists treat will have a visual problem among other impairments. There is a large vocabulary of terms used to describe visual difficulties, with which it is helpful for occupational therapists to familiarise themselves. The British Orthoptic Society has published a glossary of these terms (The British Orthoptic Society, 1979).

However slight the visual problem may appear to be, it should never be disregarded, for seemingly minor impairments may affect a child's performance during occupational assessment and treatment sessions and thus the therapist's estimate of his abilities. There are numerous causes of imperfect visual acuity, some of which will persist through life and others may resolve as the child matures. A child who lacks binocular vision, suffers from strabismus, an accommodation defect or nystagmus will have visual problems, as will those who have poor ocular movements of visual field defects.

Hemiplegia

This condition is often accompanied by a visual field defect which may result in the loss of as much as half the fields (hemianopia). The loss may be on the same side as the hemiplegia and it is important to appreciate that the lack of attention given to toys presented to that side is not only a result of the motor deficit (Pritchard, 1969). The child must be made aware of his hemiplegic side by encouraging its use to stabilise toys and equipment for bilateral activities and for making hand prints, etc. While the child must be encouraged to adopt a symmetrical posture he will also need to be reminded that when engaged in activities sitting at a table he must be sure to examine the whole of his work area. This point is important when he is doing tasks such as completing large formboards or working on a large drawing or painting when his inattention to certain areas may be mistakenly interpreted as inability.

Peripheral vision and tunnel vision

These defects may severely limit a child's visual fields or cause only relatively minor difficulties. The occupational therapist must understand the extent of the visual limitation and the effects which it will have on the child's abilities. Those who are able to use only the periphery of their visual fields and those whose vision is limited to the central fields will need to use head movements to compensate for the deficiencies. It may be necessary to encourage some to attend to previously neglected areas in order for them to learn efficiently from their environment and objects within it. These children should be taught to use head movements to ensure that they have scanned the whole of the working area. They will need more time in which to do this than the child with full visual fields. Special care should be taken to ensure that during assessment, treatment, home and school life children with such visual defects make the best use of residual vision and that parents and teachers understand the nature and implications of the impairment.

Nystagmus

This repetitive oscillatory movement of one or both eyes may be one of a number of impairments from which a child suffers. The direction of the oscillatory movement may be horizontal, vertical, rotary or retractory. The degree of nystagmus may vary according to the direction of gaze or the distance of the point of fixation. Many children with nystagmus will discover for themselves the angle of gaze at which there is minimal oscillation and thus hold their head in an asymmetrical posture. Before working towards head symmetry the therapist should ascertain the reason for the child's asymmetrical head position; while symmetry is desirable in children with neurological deficits, such as cerebral palsy, it may not be suitable for a child with nystagmus who is trying to minimise the effects of his condition. Many children with spina bifida, especially when it is associated with hydrocephalus, suffer from nystagmus.

Visual scanning

This is involved in a number of skills which the occupational therapist will wish to develop. Many activities will include visual sequencing, objects to scan in order, colour sequences to remember, words or symbols to recall in sequence. Such tasks require regular visual scanning in a particular direction as well as the perception of the relationship of each element to the others. Care should be taken to ensure that perception is not confused with visual scanning because it is often difficult to discriminate between the two. It is sometimes effective to alter the direction of the sequence of elements, though not the sequence itself, for some children have more regular visual saccades in some directions than others.

Binocular vision

This may not be achieved for a variety of reasons and without it the child will have difficulty with the appreciation of depth and distance. These skills are vital for effective functioning within the environment. Defective depth perception will make negotiating stairs, particularly unfamiliar ones, hazardous because the child will not know how much to raise or lower the foot. It will be difficult for him to estimate the height of the chair seat or an obstacle he wishes to step over. Similar problems arise because of difficulty judging distance. One particularly hazardous situation is crossing a road when the speed as well as the distance of approaching vehicles must be judged. The combination of these difficulties along, with motor deficit may create additional problems at both a gross and fine motor level. Difficulty with the precise manipulation of objects in relation to each other will be increased and the child confined to a wheelchair will have problems manoeuvring it around and between obstacles. Occupational therapists are particularly concerned with these areas of development and so she should be aware of the visual problems which may cause such deficits.

HEARING

As with other sensory impairments, hearing loss may be slight or severe, it may involve all sound frequencies or, more usually, a range of the frequencies which are normally audible. A typical example is that of children suffering from athetiod cerebral palsy who often have normal or near normal hearing for the lower frequencies and a considerable loss for the middle and higher frequencies which are necessary to hear speech. A high frequency loss makes hearing consonants particularly difficult.

It is often difficult to make an accurate assessment of the hearing of a young child and it becomes even more so if the child has additional impairments which preclude the movements which a normal child would make in response to sounds. Young babies usually stir to a new sound and slightly older ones will turn to the direction from which they hear the sound. A baby with a severe motor impairment may not be able to respond in this way. This type of testing, sounds in free field, provides only a fair estimate of the frequencies of sound which can be heard. It is only possible to make a completely accurate assessment of useful hearing with a child who is able to co-operate with the tester in some way, usually by some movement when a sound is heard. In this way it is possible, with a co-operative child, to produce an accurate audiograph of his hearing. There will be occasions when the occupational therapist will be able to devise a toy or suggest a movement with which a child is able to respond to audiometry. She will be aware of the types of activity which are best suited to a particular child and will be able to adapt such play to provide a response to sound during a hearing test.

Hearing loss can cause serious impediments to communication which may become the most serious handicap from which a multiply handicapped child suffers. 'The communication difficulty may finally prove to be the greatest disability of all in cerebral palsied people. Without adequate communication social life, even at a most elementary level, is impossible' (Fisch, 1969, p. 55). Dr Fisch goes on to explain that it is the comprehension element of communication, the understanding and knowledge of language which imposes the greater handicap, rather than the inability to communicate by means of spoken language.

Considerations when treating the child with impaired hearing

1. If the child with hearing impairment is to gain the greatest benefit from his sessions with his occupational therapist he must be seated in a good position so he can see her face and gestures clearly. The therapist should sit opposite the child so that he can see both her and any equipment he is using.
2. The child should have his face at the same level as the therapist's, which should be well illuminated since communication involves more than the spoken word. The child will glean much information from the expression on the therapist's face, and how she holds and moves her head.
3. The method of communication with the deaf child will not usually be decided by the occupational therapist alone; the staff of the audiology department, speech therapists and, if appropriate, the policy of the local education authority will influence the methods to be used. The occupational therapist should familiarise herself with whichever method is used, and practise the skills so that she may communicate freely with the child.

TOUCH

Most of our waking and sleeping hour involve the use of the sense of touch. Part of the body is at all times in contact with another part of itself or some element of the environment. Much of this contact is not consciously acknowledged but, nevertheless, the sensations thus received are perceived and allow appreciation of self, position of self and relationships to other objects.

Children in whom one of the other senses is deficient often rely to a greater extent on the sense of touch. Children who are blind or who have a severe visual impairment are often severely delayed in their motor milestones. If the development of gross motor skills is considered chronologically the usual sequence is from lying — when a large proportion of the body surface is in contact with a solid surface — through sitting to standing and walking — when only the soles of the feet or foot are in contact with a hard surface. A normal child uses his visual sense to monitor his position in space and relationships to objects in his environment. A child who suffers from a severe visual handicap is, of course, unable to do so and it seems that to compensate for this deficiency he keeps as large a proportion as possible of his body surface in contact with a hard surface; hence the apparent delay in motor milestones.

An area of special tactile sensitivity is the mouth. All babies pass through a stage of mouthing objects which they hold in their hands. By this means they learn many details of the nature of objects, their roughness, smoothness, hardness, softness and their taste. Children who have impaired manipulation continue mouthing objects long after the age at which most children have ceased to do so. Could it be that this phenomenon is not simply a developmental delay but a means whereby these children who find manipulation difficult discover the nature of objects which others would do by manipulation? It could be speculated further that such children are also handicapped by the fact that they are exploring objects orally rather than manually and are therefore impeded in the co-ordination of simultaneous tactile and visual skills — eye-hand co-ordination. These suppositions raise questions for the occupational therapist about her treatment of such children. Should mouthing be discouraged in the child who has impaired manipulation and efforts be made to encourage the development of effective manipulation, or should the child be allowed to mouth at will in order to utilise his most sensitive means of touch? Perhaps the most realistic approach is to differentiate between mouthing as a ritualistic self-stimulating habit and the purposeful mouthing which take place to discover the qualities of an object.

The hands are the parts most commonly associated with the sense of touch. The normal child finds it difficult to restrain himself from touching. How often is a parent heard to rebuke a child in terms such as, 'Look with your eyes not your hands!' Most children and, in fact adults too, find 'looking' with their hands irresistible. Adults will want to know the feel of material which looks beautiful or to hold an interesting piece of pottery. The childlike urge to experience the wetness of water or to 'feel' to see if the sign 'wet paint' is true is irresistible as is the desire to touch any visual attractive object. The combination of vision and touch reveals so much information.

Tactile skills

For some children the actual sensation of touch is diminished. Many children who suffer from hemiplegia have reduced sensation on the affected side which can be demonstrated in clinical tests, but also less formally in a therapeutic setting in combination with tests of perception of individual fingers (Kinsbourne, 1968) and comparisons of object recognition in the affected and unaffected hands.

Test of two point discrimination

These tests are used to ascertain the child's ability to distinguish two points on the skin where he is being touched. Such tests are, of course, impossible with very young children and older ones who are unable to respond reliably.

Finger gnosis

The ability to recognise the finger which is being touched when vision is excluded. Again the child must be able to indicate his responses reliably. The child is asked to place his hand on a flat surface, palm downwards. His hand is screened from his view with a piece of heavy paper or card. A finger is chosen at random and touched, the screen is removed and the child is asked to indicate which finger was touched. All the fingers are tested in random order. Those which the child fails to identify are retested. It is common to find difficulty distinguishing between the middle and ring fingers (see Figure 4.3).

Figure 4.3: Testing finger gnosis

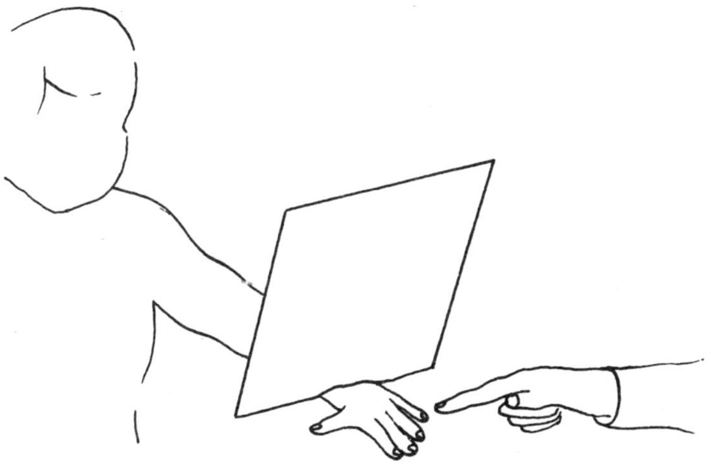

Stereognosis

The ability to recognise objects by touch may be tested by presenting the child with a selection of small common objects which have been sewn into small bags. The child is asked to feel each bag and say what he thinks it contains. The bags should be made of soft closely woven material which has a small distinct pattern printed on it. It has been found that plain material allows the child to recognise the object contained in the bag by its outline whereas a patterned fabric helps obscure it. According to the situation the objects may be explored with one or two hands. Some children with expressive language difficulties will be unable to name the objects though they recognise the contents of the bag. For such children an array of objects identical to those contained in the bags will allow them to point to the one which they have felt in the bag. It has been found that children find it much easier to indicate the objects recognised in the bags by pointing to a similar one than by naming them because the former method allows them to see a limited number of possibilities whereas the latter makes the choice almost infinite. The occupational therapist, therefore, should note carefully the method which the child uses to identify the objects.

Suitable objects to place in bags to test stereognosis are: spoon, pencil, coin, door key, small toy car, comb, and toothbrush. The selection of objects presented will depend on the age and experience of the child.

Both the above tests contain elements in addition to touch, namely perception of body image when recognising fingers, and manipulation and shape perception when recognising objects. Other tests of manipulation and perception should be used before diagnosing problems with the sense of touch.

The feel and the child's grip of an object

A defective sense of touch will affect the ability of the child to use his fine motor skills because the type and strength of grip exerted upon an object depends to some extent upon how it feels. A ball which feels hard and ungiving will be gripped in a different way to one which feels soft and squashes easily. Lack or impairment of this appreciation impedes appropriate grip. It is uncomfortable and could be hazardous to grip a very rough or jagged surface too firmly. Objects which are slippery need to be gripped gently if they are not to shoot out of the hand.

The effect of hand skills on tactile experience

The child who has impaired manipulation is also likely to have less experience of tactile sensation. Hands which are involuntarily flexed because of spasticity, those with impaired movement due to JCA or arthrogryphosis, those whose power of movement is impaired by muscular atrophy or muscular dystrophy, the hands of the child suffering from spina bifida which are used for propping, will all be deprived of sensory experience. Children who are not able to move within their environment will be deprived of sensory experience unless they are brought within their reach. For all such children many of the experiences common to the normal child are unattainable. Their hands have never reached inside a packet of cereal to crush the crisp flakes and their hands have never been blackened by the rough soil of raw unwashed potatoes. Few will have smashed an egg and felt the sliminess of the contents or played with stones or sharp gravel. Special thought should be given to thousands of sensory experiences of normal childhood and efforts made to incorporate at least some of them into the lives of children who are unable to make these discoveries for themselves.

TASTE AND SMELL

These two senses are very closely related: the person who suffers from an impaired sense of smell will complain that he is unable to taste his food. It is well known that the sense of smell is more acute in animals than in human beings and that the acuteness of both taste and smell diminish with age. Experiments have been undertaken to isolate the four types of taste and the smells which may be appreciated (Corso, 1967) but little has been written about the olfactory and gustatory senses of children with continuing impairment.

The blind or deaf/blind children will back up knowledge obtained from the perceptions of his intact senses by taste and smell. The appreciation of the roundness and texture of an orange will be augmented by its characteristic smell (Freeman, 1975). The sense of taste may cause extra feeding difficulties for children suffering from cerebral palsy; sharp tastes may elicit bite or gag reflexes. The occupational therapist will be able to explain this additional cause of feeding problems and suggest less provocative foods for the child.

Despite the paucity of literature on the special uses of taste and smell for the child with continuing disability, their utilisation should not be dismissed, particularly in the areas of compensating for other deficient senses.

5

Assimilating Information from the Senses

All fact-collectors, who have no aim beyond their facts, are one-story men. Two-story men compare, reason, generalize, using the labours of the fact-collectors as well as their own. Three-story men idealize, imagine, predict; their best illumination comes from above, through the skylight.

Oliver Wendell Holmes Sr, The Poet and the Breakfast Table (1872)

Input from any of the senses is of little practical use unless it is interpreted by the brain. An object is held in the hand, it is gripped according to its shape, its texture and resiliance, the eye regards it, senses its colour, its edges and the light it reflects. A person realises that the object sensed by the hand is the same one appreciated by the eye — hand and eye are co-ordinated. The object is perceived as a ball; it is recognised as belonging to the same category as many similar objects perceived in the past. It may be the same ball that has been regarded and felt many times in the past; it is remembered as such and the verbal symbol 'ball' may be attached to it.

This is the description of a process which is carried out many times each day, a process apparently so simple that it is over in a trice and rarely attracts any comment. The process of appreciating the environment and the objects it contains takes place automatically and effortlessly for most people. The perception of sensory input — recognition, insight, understanding, common sense — is the key to learning of any kind, yet comparatively little is known about it and it is extremely difficult to separate from sensory input and motor output. The process of perception is further complicated by memory, attention, motivation, concentration and distraction.

Much of the study of perception has been undertaken with people who have suffered traumatic brain damage (Blakemore, 1977; Williams, 1970). In such cases it is possible to study the pre- and post-morbid perceptual function. Information gained from such research can often be applied to the study of perception as a developmental process.

BODY IMAGE

Perception begins with knowledge of self which is often referred to as 'body image' or 'body consciousness'. This involves knowledge of self via a variety of sensory input channels, often more than one sensory input being required to form a percept. A young baby lying supine observes an object which appears in and then disappears from his field of vision. As the object appears and disappears he receives proprioceptive stimuli from the joints of his shoulder and arm. He perceives that the object belongs, is attached to himself, that he is looking at and perceiving the movement of his own arm and hand. Eventually one hand will grasp the other and he will perceive tactile information about the contact including touch, pressure on joints and skin and perhaps slight pain. The same child will, one day, see two similar objects which appear and disappear above the horizon of his tummy, by similar processes involving sight, touch and proprioception he will realise that these objects, his feet, are also part of self. Using a variety of sensory channels the infant builds a perfect image of self. He will learn his own size, his width, his girth and the length of his reach.

These abilities continue despite the constantly increasing size and changing proportions of the child (Sinclair, 1969). It has been empirically suggested by some who are in constant contact with growing children that at times of rapid growth body image is imperfect until the new image has been learned. This has been put forward as an explanation of the temporary clumsiness of some children at the time of growth spurts.

Children know without measuring themselves against a space whether or not they are able to pass through it; they automatically turn sideways if this is necessary without any visual reference to self, only the space being visually measured. They know without checking how far they can reach with an outstretched arm, when their body will also need to be extended, and when it will be necessary to move the whole of their body in order to reach a desired object. They can make fairly accurate estimates of the height of their reach standing on tiptoes with arm extended and they can decide without measuring when they will need a stool or stepladder to reach an object. The normal child knows himself extremely accurately.

Observing the child's appreciation of body image

It is easier to observe defects of body image than it is to test for them formally. However, the child may be observed in a series of situations which require appreciation of body image:

1. The child could be asked whether he considers he could pass between two chairs or similar objects placed less than the width of his body apart without disturbing them.
2. Could he pass beneath a plank raised a few inches from the floor?
3. Could he reach and grasp an object without moving from his chair? By holding an object for the child to reach in various positions the occupational therapist may judge if the child has a reasonable idea of the reach of his trunk and arm (see Figure 5.1).
4. By asking a child who is standing to stretch, reach and grasp an object held above his head the child's appreciation of his total length may be assessed.

Such tasks could be graded and the results recorded to provide a profile of a child's knowledge of his own body image.

With any assessment of the appreciation of body image other elements are involved:

1. The child is required to move, therefore motor organisation and movement are involved.
2. Equipment such as chairs and planks are used so that the child can demonstrate his appreciation of the position in space of these objects and his own spatial relationship to them.
3. There must be the involvement of language comprehension or at least the ability to imitate gesture.
4. The ability to name parts of the body should not be confused with appreciation of body image for verbal labels may be learned by rote despite defective body image.

Figure 5.1: Observing the child's appreciation of his own body image

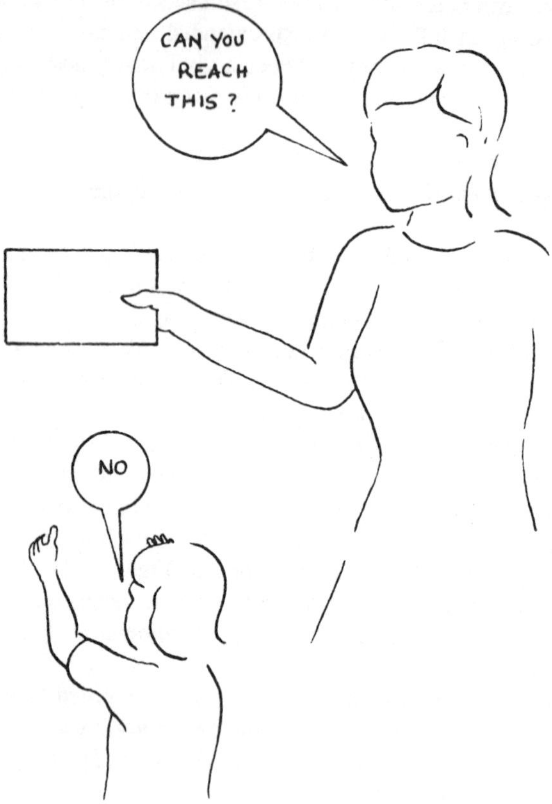

Games which draw the child's attention to his body image

1. Touch different parts of the child first with the child looking at the part being touched then with eyes closed so that he recognises by touch the part on which he feels pressure.
2. 'Drive' a small car over the child's body to draw his attention to various body parts, their relationship to each other and their size. Provide a commentary of where the car is being 'drive', and later ask the child to provide the commentary.
3. Draw around the child on a large chalkboard placed on the floor ensuring that he can feel the progress of the hand holding the chalk. Later when the child is no longer on the chalkboard, he is able to

Figure 5.2: Drawing round a child on a floor chalkboard to reinforce his appreciation of body image

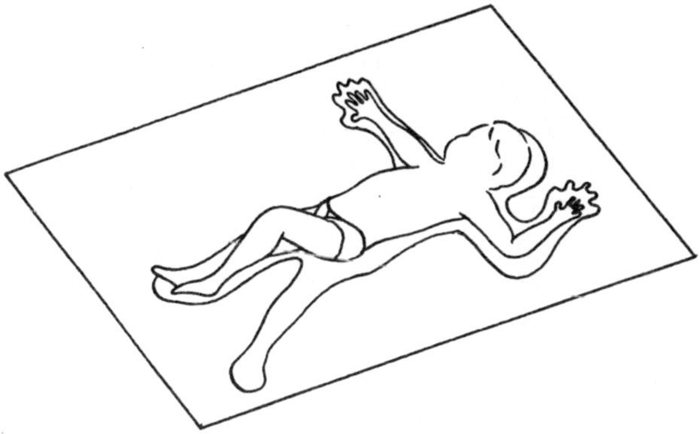

discuss the overall size of the outline and relative sizes of the body parts (see Figure 5.2).

4. Bathtime is ideal for reinforcing body image. The naked child being washed and dried, or washing and drying himself, provides visual and tactile input regarding body parts. It is a time when parents become the child's ideal therapists since body parts may be touched and examined in a very natural situation. Such therapy is part of the normal daily routine.

5. Singing games about body parts help to reinforce body image, e.g. 'Head, Shoulders, Knees and Toes', and 'Ockey, Cockey'.

POSITION IN SPACE AND SPATIAL RELATIONSHIPS

Closely related to body image are the abilities to appreciate position in space and spatial relationships. These spatial skills are important both with regards to self and objects in the environment. They also play a part at a very fine level in the acquisition of literacy and graphacy.

Normally position in space is appreciated without it being consciously recognised. Information about position in space reaches the brain via sensory receptors of touch, pressure and proprioception which transmit messages regarding body parts in contact with solid surfaces; for example, the soles of the feet in contact with the floor in standing, or the thighs in contact with a chair in sitting. Proprioception provides information about position in space in two ways — the kinesthetic and vestibular systems. Kinesthesis involves the sensitivity of body parts to movements by receptors situated in joints, muscles and tendons. The vestibular system, which is situated in the labyrinth of the inner ear, is sensitive to bodily movement in space of the body as a whole (Corso, 1967, pp. 148–51; Nathan, 1969, pp. 81–7). Usually these processes take place without conscious recognition. A change in position takes place without reference to the previous position.

Children who have spatial difficulties appear clumsy or lack grace in both posture and movement. They are often unable to grade movements and reactions. Behavioural and emotional difficulties may be superimposed on the perceptual ones. In the classroom these children often attempt to cover up their difficulties by becoming the 'class clown' or alternatively by becoming withdrawn and reluctant to attempt activities in which they fear failure. They are often the last child to be chosen to take part in team games because they are unable to react quickly in response to the actions of others and are usually abysmally poor at ball games. There is no therapy that will transform them into athletes though their spatial skills and posture can be improved by programmes of treatment which concentrate on these skills.

Suggestions to include in programmes to improve spatial skills

1. Obstacle courses comprising objects to pass over, under, around, along and through (see Figure 5.3).
2. The therapist adopts a posture which the child copies.
3. Using a mirror in which the child may monitor his position.
4. The child is presented with a series of pin men drawn on large cards. He attempts to copy their positions (Kephart, 1960) (see Figure 5.4).
5. Games which include references to body part and movements, e.g. 'Simon Says', and hand rhymes like 'Here's a Church'.

Kicking, throwing and catching a ball require accurate eye-foot or eye-hand co-ordination which in turn require good body image and spatial skills. The co-ordinated hand and eye, for example, requires the eye to monitor the object being manipulated by the hand. The eye does not monitor hand movements; the hand must manipulate without the need for visual monitoring. Catching a ball successfully includes the eye watching the approach of the ball, its distance from the hands and the speed at which it is travelling. The

Figure 5.3: An obstacle course to improve spatial skills

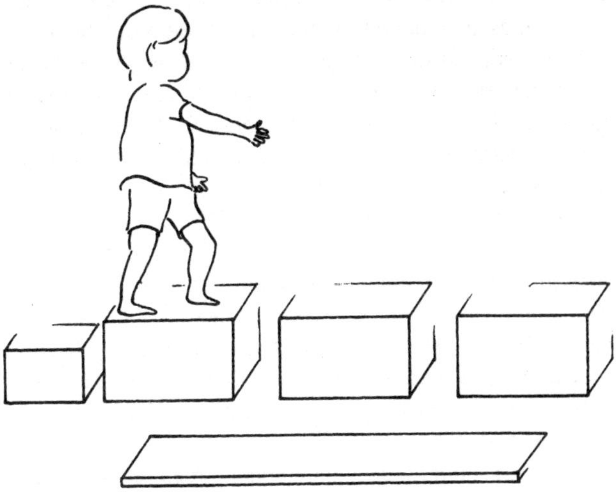

Figure 5.4: Copying the positions of pin men to improve appreciation of position in space

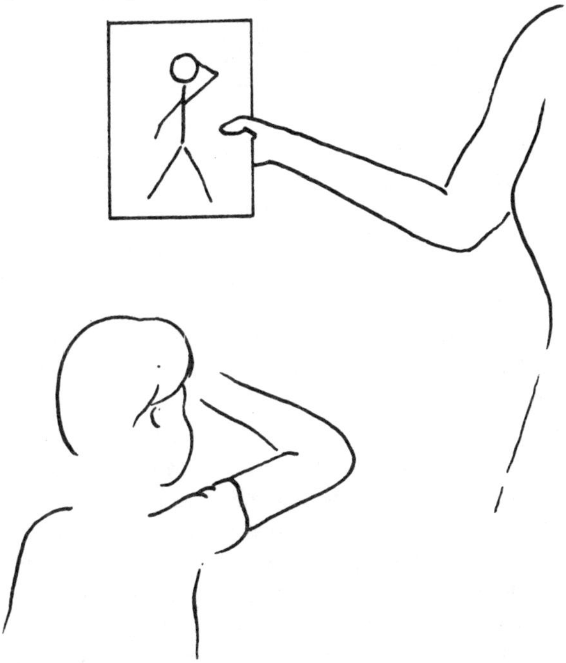

hands must be placed in a suitable position in readiness to receive the ball, their position being constantly adjusted according to the direction from which the ball is thrown so that accurate contact will be made between hands and ball. All these adjustments must be made without visual monitoring. Thus catching a ball, particularly where swift reaction is needed in response to the actions of another child, is a difficult task for the child with body image problems and spatial difficulties.

Suggestions for improving ball skills

1. Begin by using a bean bag because it is easier to catch than a ball.
2. Practise the position in space of the hands until the child knows where they are without visual monitoring and so is free to watch the flight of the ball.
3. First use a large ball which has a matt surface, gradually progressing to small balls (see Figure 5.5).
4. Before attempting to throw check the child's ability to release the ball.
5. Practise direction of throwing by using a box or bin to throw the ball into. Use balls of various sizes, weights and densities so that the child has to gauge the power required to throw the ball into the box. Move the box so that it is necessary to throw the ball further and in a variety of directions.

Children who had difficulty with throwing and catching will usually fare better at solitary sports where there is no need to respond to the actions of other people. They will cope better at bowling than batting in cricket and enjoy sports such as golf, archery and darts where there is no time element in arranging the body prior to making shots. These points should be discussed with parents so that they do not have unrealistic aims for their children and may guide them towards activities in which they are likely to meet with a fair degree of success.

Independent dressing may be particularly difficult because the task requires perception of body image, ones own position in space and that of the garments to be put on, together with complex percepts of the relationships of self and garments. The acquisition of an acceptable level of independent dressing may require the skill to be broken down into small components and processes repeated many times. Parents will appreciate advice on the purchase of suitable garments and the discreet marking of them to help the children

Figure 5.5: A large ball with a matt or textured surface is easier to catch than a shiny, small one

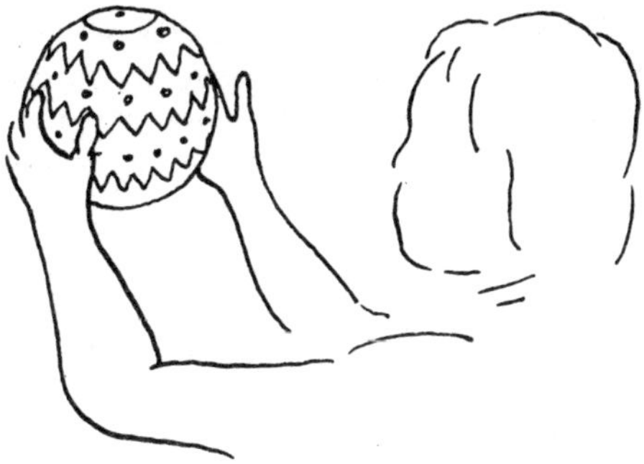

find top and bottom, back and front. For some children, particularly those with a degree of mental handicap, teaching by backward chaining is an effective method.

Often these children have few friends because of their inappropriate actions; spatial difficulties may result in an intended friendly arm round the shoulder of a classmate becoming a smack in the eye! Some children have an apparent inability to grade any motor activity including voice production. They have difficulty modulating the voice so that they either speak very quietly, almost in a whisper, or very loudly. The ability to grade the loudness of their voice may take much practice and always require conscious effort. There are children in whom the same type of problem also involves emotional reaction such as laughing and crying. The effect may appear to be similar to emotional liability when in fact the problem is one of grading reaction. There are children who have body image and spatial difficulties who either laugh uncontrollably or not at all. Similarly, when sad or miserable they find it impossible to grade their weeping according to the degree of misery they are feeling. These inappropriate displays of emotion add to their unpopularity with their peers, their reactions appearing odd to them.

Body image and spatial difficulties often coexist with other problems which may be sensory or involve other areas of perception and motor skills. The clumsy child who is at the lower end of the range of physical ability — which spans from highly agile and athletic to completely lacking grace, possibly minimally cerebral palsied — is most likely to have a number of difficulties. Each difficulty would be of little significance if it existed alone but in combination with others can cause considerable problems for the child.

Similar symptoms are often part of the more serious syndromes such as spina bifida and cerebral palsy. Children who suffer from spastic cerebral palsy, including hemiplegia, are more likely to experience such difficulties than those whose symptoms include athetosis (Foley, 1969, pp. 42–3). It is important to identify these difficulties so that differentiation may be made between motor and perceptual problems and the appropriate treatment administered.

At a gross level it is possible to observe these problems in the child who uses a wheelchair: although he may have the motor ability to control the appropriate type of chair he may, in fact, be unable to do so because he lacks an appreciation of his own position in space and his relationship to other objects — in this case himself in his wheelchair, the furniture in the room and limiting factors such as the size of doorways. As the child approaches adulthood it may be perceptual difficulties not motor problems which prevent him from successfully driving a car (Holgate, 1985). It is frequently these 'unseen' impairments which create the most insurmountable problems; motor impairments are often visible and perceived by both medical and lay people, and sensory deficits may be diagnosed accurately, particularly since the advent of equipment capable of recording the brain's response to sensory input. The analysis of perception — the brain's ability to rationalise sensory input — remains the most difficult function to analyse and remedy.

Case note

Jeremy was referred by his school medical officer to a child development centre during his first year in junior school because he was having severe difficulties with handwriting. He was assessed by the occupational therapist who discovered that his problems were of a general perceptual and motor nature involving all levels of activity.

1. He lacked appreciation of his own size and shape.
2. His appreciation of his position in space and his relationship to objects in his environment was defective.
3. He had difficulty planning movements particularly when those movements had several elements.
4. His balance was poor because he had difficulty shifting his centre of gravity as he adopted different positions.
5. He had a poor sense of rhythm.

His occupational therapist worked first at a gross motor level before concentrating on the symptom for which he had been referred — his handwriting.

Treatment techniques

1. Drawing round him with chalk on a floor chalkboard, discussing the part which was currently being outlined, and the size and shape of the completed silhouette.
2. Asking him to copy postures adopted first by his therapist, using a mirror to check his own posture.
3. Asking him to copy the postures of pin men which had been drawn on large pieces of card.
4. He repeated series of movements, e.g. two hops followed by two jumps, step right, step left, two steps forward. The importance of performing these movements slowly and rhythmically was stressed.
5. He was taught how to transfer his weight whilst swaying and later balancing on one leg. He held his therapist's hands while she performed these movements so that he could feel the transfer of her weight.
6. He was shown how to perform movements slowly at a regular tempo rather than rushing into movements as he tended to. Music was used to reinforce rhythm. Jeremy's parents were present for his twice weekly treatment sessions and practised the activities with him at home for a few minutes each day. Though he will never excel at Physical Education and games his posture and control of movement is greatly improved. When his occupational therapist turned her attention to his handwriting there was already some degree of spontaneous improvement.

FORM CONSTANCY

It is not until infants are about one year old that they appreciate the constancy of concrete objects (Vernon, 1971, pp. 21–2). Before that time, an object which is removed from sight has disappeared for ever as far as the infant is concerned. The infant does not search for an object which he has dropped from his hand; he is surprised to rediscover an object which has been covered. At about one year of age he learns that objects have a permanency, and that they still exist despite not being able to see them. He demonstrates this by searching for objects which have disappeared from view.

At about the same time the infant begins to appreciate that any three dimensional object has many aspects, whereas previously, objects were recognised only when presented in his field of vision in a familiar position. Vernon cites the example of a baby of nine months given his feeding bottle with the teat facing away from him. The infant did not reach for the bottle presented at this unfamiliar angle because he did not recognise it as his bottle (Vernon, 1971). As the infant's manipulative and hand-eye co-ordination skills mature he is able to alter their position and thus view different aspects of them, learning that an object remains the same despite its varying appearance.

Children who have motor deficits are not free to manipulate objects and so are limited in their experience of viewing them from a variety of aspects. Many have impaired locomotion and spend a large part of their day in a limited number of positions which limit their views of their environment and the objects in it.

Form constancy experience for the immobile child

1. Change the child's view of his environment frequently.
   (a) Let the child be on the floor for short spells.
   (b) Alternate spells in his positioning chair with time in a higher chair so that he may observe kitchen and other household equipment from above.
   (c) Change his position so that he can benefit from viewing his environment from prone, supine, side-lying and, if he has a standing box, from an erect position.
2. Change the position of objects in his environment.
   (a) Present him with familiar toys from different angles, e.g. his teddy bear may be presented face, back or feet first.
   (b) Have him in the room when it is being cleaned so that he sees furniture moved from its normal positions and thus its different aspects (see Figure 5.6).

FIGURE-BACKGROUND DISCRIMINATION

Being able to pick out the pertinent object or sound from a background, which may be very complex, is a fundamental perceptual skill. In both modes it is important to discriminate between a purely visual or auditory inability and a perceptual one. Poor visual acuity may make it impossible to discern some ill-defined figures from particularly complex backgrounds when there is only a small

Figure 5.6: An immobile child seeing his living room furniture from different angles while the room is being cleaned

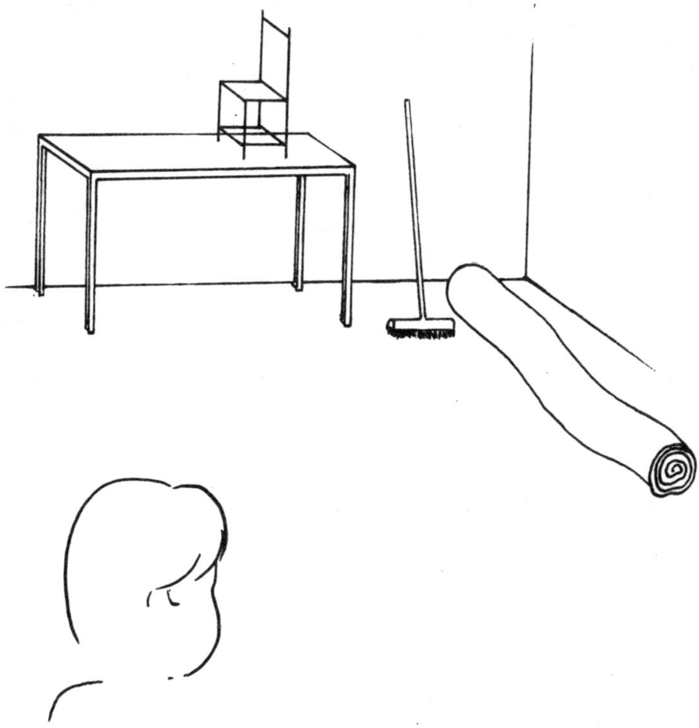

difference in the light reflective qualities of the figure and the background. Similarly poor depth perception due to lack of effective binocular vision may preclude figure-background discrimination especially if the colour intensity of the figure and the background are similar.

Figure-background discrimination — visual mode

There are children who, despite adequate vision, are unable to pick out relevant figures from backgrounds. In a normal domestic or educational setting these children have great difficulty fixating on relevant objects in their environment. They may be observed as lacking concentration, being easily distracted and flitting from one object which momentarily interests them to another.

Suggestions to help children with visual figure-background difficulties

1. Modify the environment so that the background contains no distractions. Only the equipment which the child is currently using should be on display.
2. There are children who prefer to be isolated from others in the classroom finding that in a quiet corner without decoration they are able to work more effectively.
3. Some children prefer to work in an area where there is a physical division between themselves and their peers (Geddes, 1976, pp. 89–94).
4. The Montessori Method (Montessori, 1965; Standing, 1957) has much to commend its use with children who have figure-background difficulty, and indeed many other types of problems. In Montessori Schools the rooms in which children work are free from distracting materials, unlike many classrooms which are decorated with examples of painting, writing and topic displays. Equipment not in use is stored out of sight in natural wood cabinets. Much of the teaching material is of natural polished wood without distracting motifs or pattern.

Figure-background discrimination — auditory mode

Most of the time people are in situations where they are simultaneously bombarded with a number of auditory stimuli, yet most are able to attend to the relevant sound. Consider the situation in a typical living room — the father may be repeatedly turning over, and folding and refolding the pages of a newspaper; there may be the sound of the rhythmical click of the mother's knitting needles; a sister may be making a Lego model and periodically raking through the box of pieces which produce the rattle of plastic on plastic. In the adjoining house a neighbour may be engaged in some noisy DIY tasks and through the open window and the sounds of cars' engines and slamming doors is audible as they are parked or driven away. The son of this household, nevertheless, is able to concentrate on the commentary of a wildlife programme on television: he has no difficulty with auditory figure-background discrimination.

In children in whom this ability is impaired learning becomes a haphazard affair. Noises which would not attract the attention of the child with normal skills, provide constant distractions. Such children frequently perform reasonably well in a one-to-one situation which is devoid of extraneous noise but find concentration in the average household environment or classroom almost impossible.

These are the two modalities in which figure-background difficulties are most frequently met although the possibility of misperception via other sensory channels should not be dismissed, for '. . . any pattern of sound, touch, taste, smell, etc. which is consciously perceived as such, must first become "figural" ' (Vernon, 1971, p. 43). Being able to discern the 'figure' from a complex background is fundamental to any perceptual task. A child who is able to do so will be described as having good concentration and not easily being distracted by other objects or movements. Conversely, a child who appears to lack concentration and is easily distracted may have a basic problem with figure-background discrimination.

INTELLIGENCE

Numerous definitions of intelligence have been suggested (Curzon, 1980, pp. 220–2) but argument continues about its precise nature and whether it really exists or is simply 'what intelligence tests test'. There are those who support the concept of a general intelligence factor (g), while others describe a number of mental faculties such as problem solving, planning ability, foresight and originality. In fact most tests of intelligence assess a range of mental abilities, the results illustrating the testee's strengths and weaknesses supporting the claim that '. . . it is more consistent with the statistical evidence to think of intelligence as fluid collection of abilities, comprising the whole mental life, though most prominently manifest in higher relational thinking' (Vernon, 1960, p. 31).

Children continue to be tested for the quantity and quality of the faculties they possess. The results of these tests are important for occupational therapists when planning treatment programmes, deciding treatment methods and setting appropriate goals; often it will be found that children who are deemed to have a general low level of intelligence will have great difficulty generalising concepts and in applying past experience to solve current problems. The subtests which are often grouped into verbal and performance skills will indicate the child's strengths and weaknesses. As is so often the case, it is of benefit for the psychologist who tests the child to collaborate with the occupational therapist in discussions about cognitive difficulties. The psychologist will be able to interpret her test results more realistically if she is aware of the occupational therapist's assessment of fine motor function which may affect the child's results on performance sub-tests, particularly if there is a time factor involved.

MOTIVATION

The best laid therapeutic plans will be thwarted if the child is not motivated to strive for success. In the absence of motivation the child will not be aroused with a desire to participate in activities, physical or cognitive, in order to reach appropriate goals and thus learn. At a very basic level he will be inattentive to stimuli and will not respond to them and his behaviour will not be changed — he will not have learned. There is no foolproof method of evoking motivation though recognition of motive-dampening and stimulating factors will help the effectiveness of the therapist's plans.

Factors affecting motivation

1. Previous success and failure have a profound effect on present motivation level. 'When people have succeeded, they tend to feel lively and elated; when they have failed, they may be depressed and apathetic. These feelings may be prolonged . . .' (Vernon, 1971, p. 189). Fear of failure or memory of past failure reduces the level of motivation. It is prudent, therefore, when testing a child's abilities for the therapist to begin at a level low enough to ensure success. This may prove to be ridiculously low in comparison with the child's actual level of ability but it is preferable for the child to complete a task with ease and ensured success; otherwise an assessment session could be marred by introducing tasks at such a level that the child feels his ability is being tested to its limits at all times. It is simpler for the therapist to apologise to the child for presenting him with a task which was far too easy than to have to rebuild his motivation after he has lost interest.
2. Goals must be appropriate to the child's abilities and means must be devised to attain those goals in a way which is meaningful, and therefore motivating, to the child.
3. Activities should be, as far as possible, appropriate to the occasion. Dressing is meaningless if it is undertaken for no other reason than practice. It is more appropriate for the child to play his part in

the process of undressing prior to entering the therapy swimming pool, which he eagerly anticipates, or to help with getting dressed again after a physiotherapy session. Ideally, the therapist should occasionally be present at the child's home, in the morning or evening, so that dressing and undressing practice is undertaken in the most normal of all situations; in addition, the therapist is able to take into account the conditions and habits which exist in the child's home environment. Parents are also able to carry over the therapist's suggestions so that they become integrated into daily life.

4. Hunger and thirst may hamper a therapy session by distracting the child's attention from the task in hand. On the other hand, this desire may be put to use by the therapist who wishes to work on independent feeding. A replete child will have little motivation to attempt to carry a spoonful of food from dish to mouth; hunger may provide that little bit of extra motivation which will result in success.

PERCEPTUAL ELEMENTS IN READING, WRITING AND SPELLING

Learning difficulties may occur in the absence of any other problem. There are children who have difficulty only with spelling — their ability to *recognise* words which they have previously encountered is normal so that reading is not impaired, but their ability to *recall* the letters and their order within a word is deficient so learning to spell will be difficult. Others have problems only with recording the written word; this may result from problems with spelling, the mechanics of handwriting, difficulty with constructing sentences or with ordering their thoughts on paper. Learning difficulties may result from a collection of seemingly minor sensory, perceptual and/or motor symptoms which affect every aspect of the child's life. A child who appears clumsy because of body image, spatial difficulties and lack of co-ordination will not excel during games and Physical Education classes, he may have taken longer than usual to learn to ride a bicycle, swim and dress independently; he may also have irregular, dysfluent, illegible handwriting and may have difficulty in recognising letters of similar shape but of different orientation such as *b/d/p* or *t/f* and in ordering the graphemes (letters) within words.

Body image

Knowledge of self and one's position in space is necessary for effective hand-eye co-ordination. In order to concentrate visually on a task being performed by the hands the eyes must be free; they cannot also be used to monitor hand movements.

Handwriting is perhaps the fine motor skill which requires the greatest accuracy and in which the hand is employed for prolonged periods making a variety of precise movements. Children who have body image and positional problems are, therefore, likely to manifest their difficulties in their handwriting. Many children are referred for occupational therapy because of poor handwriting. Often this is only one symptom of an impairment which includes perceptual difficulties on all gross and fine motor activities. The occupational therapist must always look further than the point of referral and examine the whole child in order to discover the basis of his difficulties. There is, however, controversy with regard to carrying over treatment of one aspect of the impairment to another. For instance, does reinforcement of appreciation of position in space at a gross level affect the faculty at the fine level manifested in handwriting? Most remedial programmes today would include treatment at both a gross and fine level. Several experiments in remediation of this type of difficulty are described by Lady Francis-Williams in her book *Children with Specific Learning Difficulties* (Francis-Williams, 1970).

Position in space

Appreciation of the position in space of graphemes in Western script is vitally important in the encoding and decoding of written language. A number of phonemes are only differentiated from others if the spatial position is appreciated. Groups of phonemes which are sometimes confused are *b/d/p*, *f/t*, *m/w* and *n/u*. Children appreciate vertical inversions, for example the differences between *n* and *u*, before they appreciate horizontal reversals, like *b* and *d*. It is considered normal for a child up to the age of seven not to appreciate horizontal reversals.

The occupational therapist should differentiate between perceptual difficulties and those caused by poor motor organisation. In the former the child will have difficulty with both the decoding of the printed graphemes (reading) and encoding them (writing). However, if motor organisation is the problem the child will not experience difficulties with reading, only with writing.

Helping the children with perceptual difficulties who confuse the orientation of letters

1. Investigate the child's general ability to appreciate position in space. Does he understand that his toys, perhaps a teddy bear or car, may be stood upright, upside down, made to face left or right? If he is presented with a horizontal array of similar animals and one of them is placed in a different orientation, does he appreciate that difference?
2. Should he have problems with these various orientations of objects let him handle them, placing each array in the same orientation. Talk to him about various positions in space and let him experiment with them.
3. Tell him stories about the letters with which he is experiencing difficulty, e.g. *m* is the letter which begins mountain and the letter looks like a mountain; *u* is the letter which begins umbrella which we use when it rains — *u* must be written so that it can hold rain. Make the subject letter into a picture to reinforce the story and thus the memory of the current orientation in the child's mind (Wendon, 1973).
4. Do not teach two letters which confuse the child in the same session; *b* should not be taught at the same time as *d*. Usually when the orientation of one of a pair of letters has been learned, the child will experience less difficulty learning the other.

Spatial relationships

In order to make sense of the written word it is necessary for the child to be able to appreciate the relationship of graphemes to each other. Many words contain a similar group of graphemes only their order differentiating one from the other. Consider such pairs of words as was/saw, spilt/split, form/from, on/no, bad/dab; the only difference between the words of each pair is the order or sequence in which the letters are arranged.

Helping the child who has difficulty with the spatial relationships of the letters within words

1. Ascertain the child's ability to cope with sequences of objects. Is he able to copy a colour sequence of bricks? Does he appreciate the relationship of the colours to each other? If he finds this difficult prepare some cards with sequences of squares of colour of the same size as the bricks and ask him to place the correct brick on each square.
2. Some children have difficulty with visual sequencing of spatial relationships but cope well with auditory sequences. Experiment to see if this is the case and if so reinforce vision with letter sounds.
3. A tactile input is the most meaningful for some children, try using plastic lower case letters of ones made from Plasticene or pipe cleaners so that the child may actually move the letters into their correct spatial relationships.
4. Where words contain digraphs or trigraphs (two or three graphemes representing one phoneme) learning the digraphs as a chunk is often helpful (Newton and Thomson, 1974). Diana Geddes has some interesting suggestions for incorporating the learning of 'chunks' into games (Geddes, 1976, pp. 63–4).

Figure-background discrimination

Some children experience great difficulty concentrating on the words they are reading within a page full of print. This is a similar problem to figure-background discrimination at a gross level. The child will not have problems reading isolated words or a sentence but will become confused when there is a large amount of print on the page. In the early stages of reading this is not usually a problem as there is little print on each page.

Helping the child with figure-background problems

1. Check with the orthoptist to ensure that the child has no optical problem with scanning.
2. The simple device of holding a strip of plain card beneath the line being read is often helpful.
3. The problem may be helped by the child moving a card in which an appropriately sized window has been cut so that only a portion

of each page is exposed at any one time. This device is only effective for the child in the early stages of reading for it does not encourage swift scanning of complete phrases and sentences.

Left-handedness and cross eye-hand preference

Despite the results of recent research (Bishop, 1980; Clark, 1970, pp. 45–9), left-handedness and crossed eye-hand preference continue to be cited as possible causes of learning difficulties. It is often noticed that children who have learning difficulties are also left-handed or have crossed eye-hand preference. *This does not infer that one is dependent on the other*. One study concluded that 39 per cent of a population of 1544 primary school age children demonstrated crossed eye-hand preference (Clark, 1970), the incidence clearly precluding that the characteristic is related to the much smaller group of children who experience learning difficulties.

The greater the number of tests of hand preference administered the less clearly defined that preference becomes because few people prefer the same hand for every type of activity. Very few people are exclusively left- or right-handed. Estimates of the incidence of left-handedness vary according to the tests being used but many recent results suggest that it is about 10 per cent (Clark, 1970; Enstrom, 1962; Lyle and Johnson, 1976) *The reason for left-handedness is more significant than the fact of left-handedness* (Bishop, 1980; Penso, 1983; Touwen, 1972).

There are left-handed people who have no choice regarding the use of that hand, obviously those with only one hand but also those with right-sided hemiplegia, those with neurological deficit of the right hand who happen to have the better function in the left hand. All those groups of people may or may not have been born with a preference for that side but trauma has decided for them that the left will produce the best functional results (Foley, 1969). For similar reasons some left-handed people appear to be particularly clumsy and hence their sinistrality is associated with their difficulties. Many of them are probably 'naturally' right-handed but choose at an early age to use the left because of a slight neurological deficit on the right; their apparently unpreferred hand, the right, will be found to be slightly less agile that the average unpreferred hand (Bishop, 1980).

Therefore, some children who prefer to use their left hand do not have problems because they are left-handed, the cause of their difficulty is in the reason for their left-handedness.

Undecided hand preference

At times, occupational therapists are asked to see children who are undecided about which hand they prefer to use. This phenomenon is observed in some children who suffer from cerebral palsy. When the function of neither hand is perfect the young child will try one then the other until he decides on the one which he feels brings the best results. Other children who have comparatively minor motor and perceptual deficits may have similar difficulties in deciding which hand to use. The problem is often highlighted when the children begins school and he is expected to use pencils and crayons regularly. Because these children have problems with fine motor skills this difficulty may be attributed to their lack of hand preference when, in fact, it is a symptom of their motor deficit. If the child's attention is not focused on the problem and he is given time to experiment and come to his own decision about handedness he will usually do so after a short time.

6

Motor Activity in Play and Independence Skills

One two,
Buckle my shoe;
Three four,
Knock at the door;
Five six,
Pick up sticks.

English Nursery Rhyme

Learning may be described as an *apparent* modification in behaviour which is more or less permanent (Curzon, 1980, p. 7). Whether that learning concerns the acquisition of a skill, knowledge or a change of attitude in order for it to be apparent, it must be observable. Usually some form of motor activity will be observed. It may be the demonstration of a motor skill such as those described in the opening lines of the Nursery Rhyme above. Demonstration of knowledge requires movement sometimes at a gross level, in other instances at a fine level as when knowledge is recorded with pen on paper, on a typewriter, electronic printer or a computer is operated. Knowledge may also be demonstrated verbally when the language areas of the brain and the muscles of articulation are involved. The learning of particular attitudes may be demonstrated in any of the above modes.

The impairment of motor ability has severe effects on life and thus the ability to demonstrate learning. Occupational therapists are concerned with purposeful activity, adaptation to life situations. The basis of these interests is the facilitation of motor response to the perception, recognition and understanding of sensory input.

Unlike the adult who has more or less reached full functional potential, there is a further dimension to consider in the child — his potentials for development and maturation have yet to be achieved. Occupational therapy should be administered in the light of this — from the point of view that potential may not be realised because of impaired function and that functional ability can improve as neurological maturation and development takes place. Treatment will be undertaken taking into consideration the broadly accepted physical and mental developmental stages (Sheridan, 1975), the fact that not all children pass through every developmental stage (e.g. not all children crawl before they walk), the current developmental level, the prognosed levels of attainment, the life style and philosophies of the children's family, the school he attends or may attend in the future.

STABILITY

Useful motor control includes not only the planning, initiation and execution of purposeful movement but also the maintainence of body posture. Any position the body assumes other than absolute prone or supine lying requires a degree of muscle tone or interaction of the antagonists and protagonists. The normal child will have the capacity to maintain the postures appropriate to his developmental level — he will be able to overcome the effects of gravity and thus maintain himself in space.

Children who have imperfect motor control may be unable to counteract the effects of gravity. Many will need to make a conscious effort to maintain their position which leaves less of the child's mental and physical abilities free for other activities. For example, the child who needs to use a great deal of effort to maintain himself in sitting will have difficulty fastening a shirt button at the same time. An infant who struggles to raise his head and maintain that position while lying prone will not be free to receive stimuli from and perceive the detail of his immediate environment. Any child who needs to concentrate on the maintainence of posture is not free to make maximum use of that position for sensory stimulation, perception or motor activity.

The child who suffers from cerebral palsy fights a constant battle with his abnormal pattern of movement and gravity. He may learn to walk sufficiently well for it to be a useful method of mobility but it may require the greater part of his conscious effort so that if he wishes to speak he must stop walking. He is unable to practise two motor skills simultaneously. Children who suffer from spina bifida frequently have poor trunk control, the severity of which will depend on the level of the spinal lesion. Hands which are used for balance and the maintainence of upright posture are not free to be used for other activities. In addition, many children suffering from spina bifida have impaired hand function which compounds their fine motor problems.

There are many other disabling conditions of childhood which impair motor function, the muscular dystrophies and atrophies, syndromes such as Down's where hypotonia causes difficulties (Hosking, 1982, pp. 83–7), myopathic and neuropathic arthrogryposis (McCarthy, 1984, pp. 175–8) and numerous others. Whatever the cause of the motor impairment the occupational therapist should consider both the function required to perform a specific skill and the motor control required to maintain the desired posture so that an activity may be undertaken. She must differentiate between activities which will improve the maintenance of posture and those which require a special posture for their execution. These considerations will allow the therapist to decide whether the child should be given maximum support so that he is free to engage himself in an activity without concern for posture maintenance or whether the purpose of the exercise is to work towards basic maintenance of posture, both being important parts of the child's treatment.

The infant whose preferred position is supine will have a very limited view of his world. This view will be further impaired should he have an asymmetrical tonic neck reflex which will, to a large extent, limit his range of vision to the left or right. In this position he will have limited ability to manipulate toys and other objects and to practise eye-hand co-ordination, for the arm will be extended on the face side (Bobath, 1966, pp. 30–2). Whilst holding an object so that he may see it, his arms will constantly need to resist gravity. He will have difficulty seeing objects which are placed near him and little ability to retrieve those which have been dropped or learning the concept of the constancy of objects (Sheridan, 1975; Vernon, 1971, pp. 21–2). His ability to learn about the nature of the world and the objects within it will be severely impaired.

Wedges

While it is important to work towards the ability to maintain a variety of positions it is also essential to facilitate postures which will encourage them. One such position which is helpful for the child with severe motor impairment is prone lying over a wedge (see Figure 6.1).

1. The child is in a good position to see his hands and the objects which he is manipulating.
2. Because his shoulders will be protracted it will be easier for him to bring his hands together in midline.
3. He can see a range of objects in his vicinity and is able to reach for them.
4. He can watch toys as they are rolled towards him or dropped toys which roll away from him.
5. The effects of gravity are reduced because he is able to touch and play with toys placed on the floor.
6. He is able to practise many of the early hand skills such as patting, raking and banging together objects held in each hand.
7. He will be encouraged to practise neck extension and bearing weight through his arms.

The size of the wedge

1. The height of the wedge should be such that the child can place his flat hands on the floor when his arms are extended.
2. The sloping side of the wedge should be the length of the child from axilla to ankle.
3. To ensure that the child's feet are placed in a mid-position between flexion and extension the point of the wedge should be removed. The size of the piece removed will be indicated by the size of the child's feet from instep to the ends of his toes (see Figure 6.1).

Gutters

For the child who does not have the ability to extend his neck, side-lying will often provide the best position for play. He may be propped in this position or placed in a foam gutter. Such a gutter is also useful for the severely impaired young child to provide a safe sleeping position where lying supine unattended is not desirable.

Figure 6.1: A foam wedge which allows the child to reach down to the floor for toys and maintain his feet in a mid position between plantar and dorsi flexion

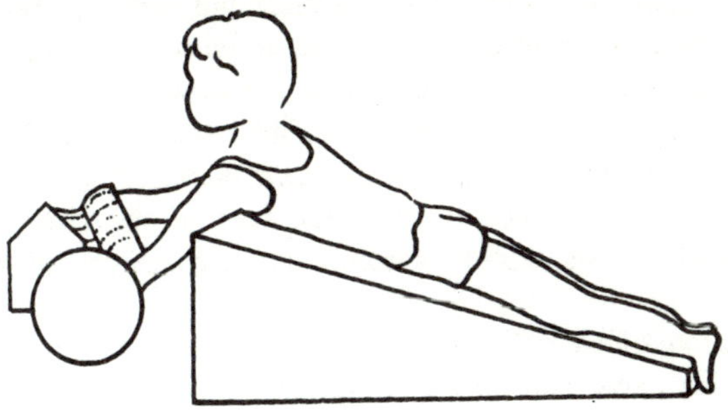

Chairs

A child who is able to sit or to be supported in this position has many advantages over the child who lies prone or supine.
1. He has an enlarged view of his environment and the possibility of partaking in a vastly increased range of activities.
2. He is in a good position to see equipment, to manipulate it and co-ordinate hand and eye.
3. Other adults and children can more easily communicate and interact with him.

All chairs should be of the simplest design possible which is at the same time effective in providing the optimum amount of control and support and being of the correct dimensions for an individual child. It may be possible to use a normal chair or to make minor adaptations to it so that it fulfils the child's needs. Wherever possible the aim should be to progress to an ordinary chair when trunk balance allows (Finnie, 1974).

Basic considerations when selecting chairs

1. The depth of the seat should support the child's thigh but should not cause pressure at the back of the knee.
2. The width of the seat should be such that if arm rests or side pieces are necessary they are in the correct position to give support.
3. The height of the seat from the floor or from the foot rest should be such that the child's knee and ankles are at right angles.
4. The height of the back of the chair should provide as much

support as is necessary.
5. Arm rests or side pieces should be at the best height for the individual child. Some children will need support up to the axilla, others will need support only to provide hip stability. Sometimes arms will only be required for the child to push against when rising to standing or to steady himself as he sits down.
6. The chair will need to be particularly stable if the child has difficulty moving smoothly from standing to sitting and vice versa.
7. Horizontal extensions to the back legs of the chair may be necessary for the child with extension spasm to prevent him tipping it.
8. The safety of the design should also be considered, especially of any moving parts, screws and wing nuts.
9. The materials from which the chair is made should be easily washable.
10. The chosen chair should be suitable for the child's home. It may be difficult to find the necessary space for a large chair in a small sitting room or kitchen. A chair which is easily portable is more likely to be used in a number of domestic situations than one which is cumbersome and difficult to carry.

Corner seats

Most children first sit and play on the floor. A corner seat, the base of which is formed by a quarter of a circle with the sides set at right angles to each other, can provide the child who is unable to sit unsupported with a play position similar to the normal child. The occupational therapist with her knowledge of seating will be able to adapt the basic principles of such a chair to the needs of an individual child (see Figure 6.2).

Adaptations to the corner seat

1. The seat may be upholstered to suit the contours of the child. Padding will make it more comfortable for the very slim child whose bones stick out, but the material used should be easy to clean, as padding creates crevices in which food and other debris is apt to collect.
2. Cross bars underneath the seat to which castors are fixed will provide the child with some mobility and allow his parents to move

Figure 6.2: A basic corner seat

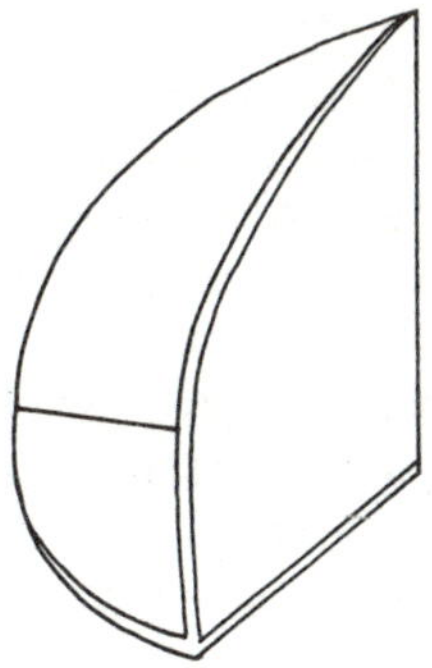

him easily to different parts of the floor.
3. For some children the shape of the corner seat provides the ideal support. A version which is raised from the floor provides a suitable position for feeding and other activities. A footrest which may be adjusted as the child grows will prolong its useful life.
4. A large tray with a lip which may be slotted on the front of the seat will provide a play area. Such a tray with a cut out will give the child added support.

A different kind of seating is required by the child who needs support to prevent the progression of deformity, as in muscular dystrophy, or to protect, as in osteogenesis imperfecta. Children who suffer from severe cerebral palsy may require this type of seating to facilitate a good working position, and a different chair when balance and trunk control is being encouraged. The supportive types of seating often makes use of individually moulded insets for chairs using thermoplastic or shapeable matrix material (Rockey and Nelham, 1984, pp. 255–73).

The child who needs support in sitting will require that support for those activities which are usually performed in this position — feeding, potty training, play and formal education.

Chairs used when the child is feeding

There is often a tendency for parents of children who are unable to support themselves in sitting to prolong the habit of feeding them on their lap in a semi-reclining position. This practice prevents the child flexing his neck which makes it difficult for him to take food actively from the spoon, encourages gagging, and hinders lip closure, chewing and swallowing.

As with many other activities, a good sitting position is a prerequisite of the formation of good eating patterns.

1. The child who has poor trunk and head control must be supported so that he feels secure and can give all his attention to the feeding process.

2. The basic principles of seating apply — the chair should be of a suitable width for the child so that lateral support is provided, and usually the height from the floor or the level of the foot rest should maintain the child's feet in a plantigrade position and the knees at right angles.

3. The hips should, if possible be at less than a right angle to encourage neck flexion and to bring the shoulders and arms forward.

4. The height of the tray attached to the chair is important, particularly if a bar or post is attached to it for the non-feeding hand to maintain extension of that arm.

5. A tray slightly higher than normal is often helpful so that the elbow of the feeding arm can be supported on it for stability.

6. Some children who suffer from cerebral palsy and others who have a limited range of joint movement cope with independent feeding if the height of the tray allows spoon feeding in only the horizontal plane.

Chairs used while the child is playing

Often the chair which is suitable for feeding will also provide a good position for play. The tray, however, should be large enough to accommodate a variety of toys and a wide range of activities.

1. A lip round the edge of the tray (except on the edge at which the child is sitting) will prevent toys being 'lost'.

2. A tray which slopes down towards the child will enable the child who finds downward gaze uncomfortable to see his toys more comfortably.

3. A non-slip surface will prevent toys rolling down an inclined tray. It will also help to stabilise toys for the child with tremor, ataxia or athetosis.

4. The colour of the tray should be a strong contrast to the colour of play materials for the child with visual problems.

5. The child who has difficulty with figure-background discrimination should have a tray without a pattern on it.

Play in childhood suggests freedom to explore and satisfy curiosity. The child who must play in a supportive chair with a tray attached certainly does not have a great deal of freedom in the lay sense of the word yet in this position he will have more freedom to indulge in play activities than in a less restricted position. This point may need to be stressed to parents and other non-professionals who may feel that such restriction is unkind.

Standing boxes

Children who are not able to stand independently at the appropriate chronological age may benefit from using a standing box or standing frame. The upright posture encourages body drainage in addition to augmenting the child's view and perception of his environment. Good positioning and appropriate support are essential to ensure extension of the hips, knees and plantigrade feet. This change of position is particularly important for the child who has little independent movement and who cannot adjust his own position. It has been found that some children have their best hand function in an upright position.

Toilet facilities

Many children who have physical and/or mental disabilities frequently have difficulty attaining bowel and bladder control, which in some results from the nature of their disabilities, and in others because normal toilet arrangements do not provide the required amount of stability and sense of security. A child who has difficulty balancing in sitting will not feel confident and relaxed on the normal potty or WC. He will need additional support in order to feel secure, the nature of which will depend on the severity of his disability.

1. Where the child has only slight instability the provision of a potty with a base broader than the top may suffice.
2. Placing the potty in the corner of the room or in the corner of a sturdy box so that the child has support on either side will give the child a sense of security. It will give a degree of trunk support to the child who cannot quite sit unsupported (see Figure 6.3).

Figure 6.3: A potty placed in the corner of a room to give the child support on two sides and make him feel secure

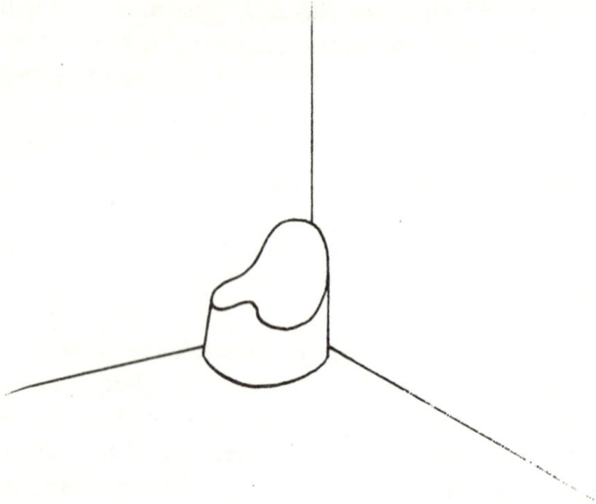

3. Wall bars as used in the Peto system of treatment will help some children to use their potty. The bars arranged down the wall should be of a diameter suitable for the child's grip and arranged 7 to 10 cm apart. The child may 'climb' down them with his hands as he bends his knees to sit on his potty, hold on to them with outstretched arms as he uses the potty and 'climb' up them with his hands as he raises to standing (see Figure 6.4).
4. Children with more severe problems will require some form of potty chair which is custom made for their needs with support at the sides back and front.

It is preferable for the older child to use the WC which, in the home situation, will usually be the same one as is used by the rest of the family. This fact should be taken into consideration when planning adaptations for the child with disabilities; they should not be so complex as to create problems for other family members. Adaptations will include those to the WC itself and, for the ambulant child, those which allow him to position himself on the WC independently.
1. The simplest adaptation is a child-size toilet seat which fits inside the proper seat, thus reducing the size of the aperture. It is ideal for any small child who is making the transition from using a potty to using the toilet as well as for small children who are slightly unstable.

Figure 6.4: Wall bars to help the child sit down on and rise from his potty

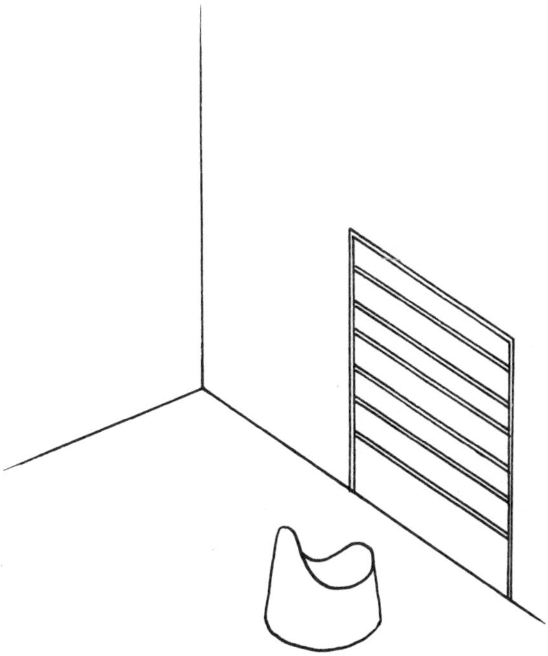

2. A grab rail on an adjacent wall will aid some children getting on and off the toilet and aid balance whilst using it. The angle at which the rails are fixed will depend on the position in which the child can best grip them. Some children have a better vertical than horizontal grip and for others the reverse is true.
3. Two shallow steps, with the treads 25 to 30 cm wide, so that it does not need to be removed when other members of the family use the toilet, and the risers 7 to 10 cm high, will provide the means for some children to use the toilet independently. A grab rail at the side of these steps provides further support (see Figure 6.5).
4. As far as possible the position of the flush handle, press button or chain should be chosen to suit the child with impairment. Placing it within reach of his 'good' hand will mean greater independence and privacy for him, a point which will become increasingly important as he becomes older.
5. The toilet paper holder should also be placed in a suitable position for the child to reach. A fitment which holds interleaved paper is

Figure 6.5: Two shallow steps and grab rail to help the unstable child to use the toilet independently

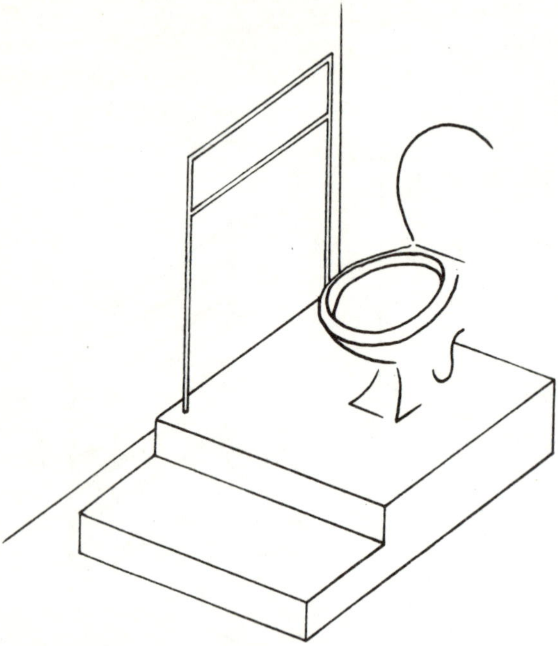

often the most suitable especially if the child is able only to use one hand. Fittings which hold a roll of paper may also be suitable if they enclose the paper except for a slot which has a serrated edge on which the paper may be torn using only one hand.

6. For the child with severe impairment a moulded seat which fits over the WC and provides support for the head, trunk and thighs with straps to maintain the position of the shoulders and pelvis may be needed.

Nancie Finnie describes a useful selection of simple toilet aids in her book, *Handling the Young Cerebral Palsied Child at Home* (Finnie, 1974).

Bathing

The ability to sit securely in the bath is important both for the child and for the adult who is bathing him. For the child to gain the maximum degree of independence in washing he may need adaptations to the bath and the surrounding area.

1. A non-slip mat in the bottom of the bath may be all that is required for the child to feel secure.

2. Grab rails will help the child with slight instability get into and out of the bath. They must be situated in the best position for the child who will be using them. Consideration must also be given to how and where they are secured. If they are fixed over the taps care must be taken that the taps are secure as the child will exert a great deal of pressure on them as he pulls himself up from or along the bath. Care should also be taken if grab rails are to be attached to the bathroom wall as often at least one wall is breeze block or similar material not suitable for the attachment of fittings which will take a lot of strain.

3. Some children require trunk support while in the bath. A canvas corner seat will often suffice. An alternative homemade solution is to use half or more of a plastic laundry basket, according to the size of the child, with holes through which his legs may pass. Because these baskets have holes in them the child is able to enjoy the sensation of water around his body. From the carer's point of view a supporting bath aid removes their need to support the child thus leaving both hands free to attend to the child's bathing needs.

4. The daily lowering the child into and lifting him out of the bath often causes permanent back injury to his carers, particularly as he increases in size and weight. One solution to this problem is a bath inset which reduces the depth of the bath and hence the depth to which the child needs to be lowered. Shower taps are a useful additional feature for rinsing when an inset is being used with an immobile child. The inset must be removed when the bath is used by another member of the family so it is important that it may be easily stored yet readily available when the child uses the bath.

5. A shower will be more suitable than a bath where a child is working towards independence and also where a child will always require some degree of help. In all cases the heat of the water must be thermostatically controlled and the pressure of water should not be affected by the opening of other water taps in the house.

(a) If the child is to be assisted in the shower there should be plenty of room for the helper to pass around the child or it will be impossible to wash the child without the helper becoming very wet. A shower head which is easily removed from its bracket is useful for rinsing the child.

(b) The child working towards independent showering will need

Figure 6.6: Shower with slatted bench to which the child may transfer from his wheelchair. The shower control and towel rail are within reach

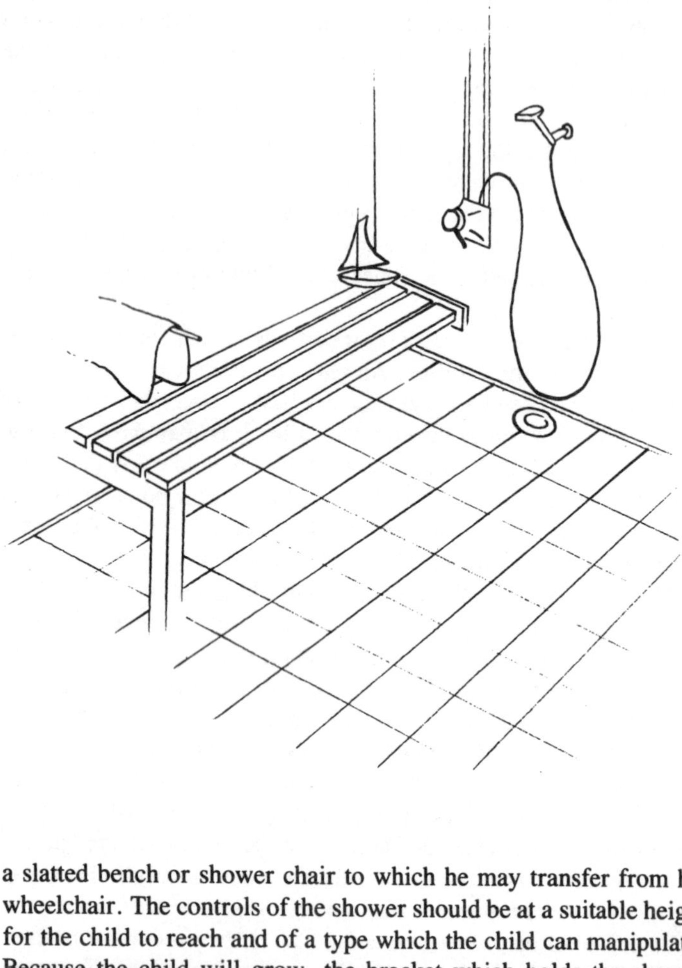

a slatted bench or shower chair to which he may transfer from his wheelchair. The controls of the shower should be at a suitable height for the child to reach and of a type which the child can manipulate. Because the child will grow, the bracket which holds the shower head should be adjustable (see Figure 6.6).

6. Of particular importance for the child working towards independence are the bathroom accessories which he will use.

(a) He will need hooks or a flat surface on which to place his clothes in a position where they will not become wet but where he may readily retrieve them.

(b) A washing mitten may be more suitable that a flannel because

Figure 6.7: A wash hand basin allows wheelchair access, a magnetic soap holder, taps and plug which are easy to manipulate

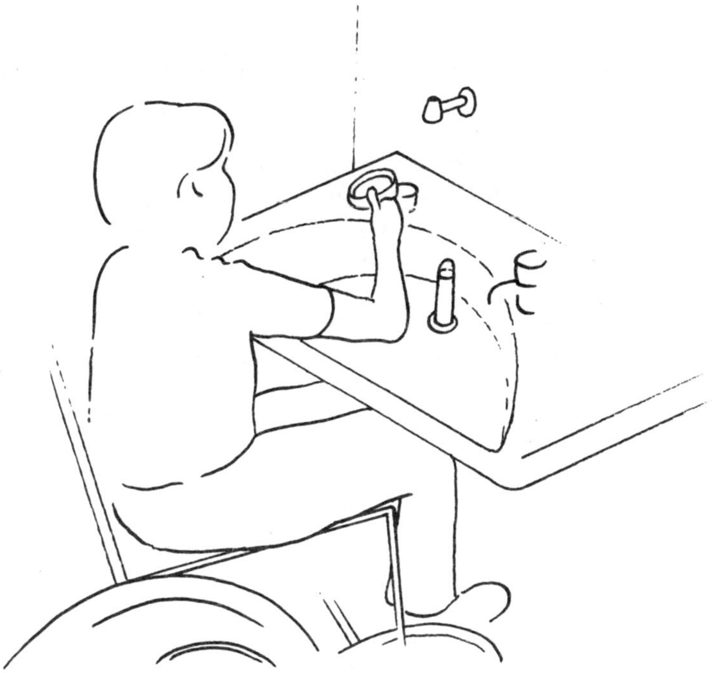

he will not loose it if he releases his grip.

(c) It may be easier for him to take hold of a piece of soap from a magnetic holder than from a soap dish (see Figure 6.7). Other children may find liquid soap in a dispenser bottle easier to manage, especially if the bottle is secured.

(d) A tablet of soap sandwiched between two pieces of 1 cm thick foam, the edges of the foam attached to each other by two rows of machine stitching, combines soap and sponge in one easily manipulated unit.

7. An electric toothbrush will help the child who has difficulty with rapid reciprocal movements to clean his teeth more effectively. A battery operated brush is safer than one which is operated by mains electricity. The disadvantage is that the batteries are usually

contained in the handle of the brush which increases both its weight and the diameter of the handle.

MOBILITY

Around the age of six months many infants become mobile, they learn to move by rolling, a couple of months later they will be able to crawl and then to creep, and between the thirteenth and fifteenth month they will usually take their first independent steps (Illingworth and Illingworth, 1984, pp. 100–19). There is variation, of course, in the ages at which children reach the various stages of mobility — some take their first steps as early as nine or ten months, others do not walk until they are 20 months or more. Not all children pass through every stage of development; some never use creeping as a means of locomotion. Often these children are bottom shufflers who usually begin to walk later than the child who creeps.

The normal child usually has some method of locomotion before he is one year old. This, of course, is a source of delight and pride to his parents and the date of his first few steps is proudly imprinted in the memories of most parents. The ability to walk is of great psychological importance to parents and the inability of many children with disabilities to do so causes much distress. Many parents feel that if their child could walk independently their problems would be largely solved. It is important that parents should be guided to see the problems of their child's lack of mobility in relation to his other skills. In reality, the ability to communicate successfully is far more important than walking ability when preparing for independent living. For the child with a severe mental handicap, walking may be the least useful skill to strive for. A child who cannot use the skill purposefully to learn and discover, who is not aware of common dangers, will require constant supervision throughout his waking hours.

Mobility immediately enlarges the world of the child, it increases the opportunity for sensory stimulation of every type. The home becomes a feast of new experiences, there are new things to see, touch, hear, taste and smell, there is heat and cold, roughness and smoothness, hardness and softness, wet and dry, etc. to investigate and examine. There are new perceptions to appreciate, of self in different positions, objects seen from various aspects, personal experience of on, under, in, behind, etc.

There are many reasons for impaired mobility — general developmental delay, abnormal neurological, muscular or joint development.

There are children who will eventually have normal mobility, those who will always need the help of equipment, such as sticks and walking frames, and those who will never be mobile except with the aid of wheelchairs or other mechanical or electronic devices.

Particularly with the older severely impaired child, his own views on his preferred methods of mobility are of paramount importance. For example, a child suffering from spina bifida may have practised walking for a number of years wearing callipers and using a rollator. He may then decide that though he is able to walk in laborious fashion it is not, for him, a practical means of mobility and so he opts for a life in a wheelchair and reserves his energies for other pursuits.

Some children, including some of those who suffer from cerebral palsy, will never be able to use walking as an effective means of mobility and will always have a wheelchair. The propulsion of a wheelchair usually depends on upper limb function unless it has been specifically adapted to be operated by some other part of the body. It is the occupational therapist who will decide the type of controls best suited to a particular child. For some children there is a choice between a manually operated chair and an electric or electronic one. A manually operated chair requires a considerable degree of effort on the part of the child. It may be desirable that the child makes this effort in order to encourage movement and development of the upper limb. On the other hand, it may not be desirable for the child to expend so much effort in the propulsion of his chair that he has little energy left for other activities.

There is a percentage of children who will only be able to operate a chair with controls which require the minimum of effort. Such children may be in the advanced stages of one of the muscular dystrophies, muscular atrophy or rarer conditions such as arthrogryposis. The occupational therapist will be involved in choosing or designing the most appropriate control system for a particular child (Harpin, 1981, vol. 6). For the child who is never expected to be independently mobile the early provision of alternative means of movement is essential since this is necessary to enlarge the child's experience, satisfy his curiosity and broaden his learning experiences.

Case note

Emma was diagnosed soon after birth to be suffering from spinal muscular atrophy and is not likely to achieve independent mobility. She has diminished muscle power and so was provided with toys which were lightweight, foam bricks instead of wooden ones and formboard rather than posting boxes, to minimise lifting.

She is a bright girl and she became more demanding of her parents' attention at home, in part because she was unable to investigate activities and objects as an able child would have done. She was provided with a 'Comet' powered chair which is controlled by a joystick which responds to the lightest pressure. Its compact rounded shape and six small wheels make it highly manoeuvreable in restricted spaces.

Emma quickly learned to operate her chair and her delighted mother reported, 'For the first time in her life she can be naughty! She "runs away" when I call her, hides behind doors and gets into all kinds of mischief in the kitchen cupboards'. Providing Emma with a means of mobility has given her freedom to learn and discover in a way which would never have been possible without it.

The parent's attitude

How do the child's parents feel about the provision of a particular piece of mobility equipment? Their co-operation is vital if it is to be of practical help for their child. The reasons for providing the aid should be discussed with the child and his parents and opportunity provided for them to air their opinions and doubts. Whenever possible the occupational therapist should visit the child at home so that decisions about self-help adaptations may be made in the light of the amount of space available and the life style of the family.

1. Will other adaptations be necessary in order for the equipment to be used? Will ramps be required or doors rehung or adapted in order for the child and his equipment to pass through.
2. Does it suit the life style of the family? An indoor chair will be under used in a family that spends a large amount of time out of doors in the garden or on camping trips.
3. Is it too large or too heavy to be easily stored in the family car? If so it may be underused or used only at the weekend when father is available to lift and manoeuvre it.

EATING AND DRINKING

Most children pass through periods when they do not eat as much as their parents feel they should or when they seem to be surviving on very limited variety of foods. Most children who have as a model parents who enjoy mealtimes as a pleasant social occasion, when a variety of foods and recipes are received enthusiastically and no undue attention paid to what and how much others eat, will eventually develop, similar eating habits. These points should be made to parents who perhaps have a child who is a little developmentally delayed and whose eating habits are giving rise to parental concern.

A basic prerequisite of eating well is being able to sit comfortably, securely and at a suitable height at the table. Whenever possible this should be the table at which all the family eat. Problems are often created by feeding a child separately from the rest of the family where all attention is focused on him and how he is coping with transferring food from plate to mouth. This habit probably began in babyhood when the child was fed by an adult and persists because he continues to have problems with eating independently. There are, of course, children who have such severe feeding difficulties that their protracted mealtimes will require the full attention of an adult. Often it will not be possible to include such children at the family meal table.

Children who have difficulty with co-ordination and who appear clumsy or lacking grace often have minor feeding difficulties which their parents may describe as being faddy. Should the occupational therapist pursue this point further and ask specifically about foods the child does and does not like she will frequently find that he does not like foods which require to be fragmented by a lateral chewing action, such as meat, apple skin, cabbage or celery. If this proves to be the eating pattern she should investigate further and watch the child eating to ascertain the quality of his lip closure and chewing pattern.

The main difficulties experienced while eating and drinking are: lip closure; chewing; swallowing; independent transference of food from plate and drink from cup. In many centres the process of disposing effectively of food in the mouth is dealt with primarily by the speech therapist, and the gross positioning of the child and the provision of suitable cutlery and crockery by the occupational therapist. In practice, of course, it is not possible to draw a definite line between the roles of the two therapists and usually it would not be expedient to do so. Ideally, there should be an overall plan regarding feeding which could include not only speech and occupational therapists but also the child's physiotherapist, who will understand the child's general pattern of movements and limitations. In the case of the child with impaired vision the orthoptist may also have pertinent suggestions to make, such as the colour of the plate the child will see most easily and the best contrasting colour from the table on which it is placed. There are occasions when feeding problems have a behavioural basis when the advice of a psychologist will be helpful.

Particularly in the case of feeding the child's parents are his best therapists and time spent teaching them the principles of encouraging good habits and independence will be most profitable. It is important, too, that when the child with feeding problems is acutely sick and is admitted to hospital that the staff on the ward are taught how to deal with him at mealtimes. Unless specially trained, nurses are used to dealing with normal children who are acutely sick and will usually welcome advice on the positioning and feeding of the child with continuing impairment.

1. Many of the principles of general positioning apply to the child who is being fed, helped to feed or feeding independently. The child's head should be well flexed because it is difficult to attain lip closure and swallowing if the neck is extended. A flexed position also tends to reduce the intensity of the gag reflex which often causes difficulty for children suffering from cerebral palsy.
2. The dish of food should be in the child's mid-line, even if he is being fed, to encourage the child to look at his food and follow its journey from dish towards mouth as well as encouraging him to maintain a symmetrical position.
3. The child should be encouraged to come forward to take food off the spoon by closing his lips around it.
4. Effective chewing can only take place if the lips are closed; if necessary the child should have help in keeping his lips closed by placing a hand under the chin and applying upward pressure.
5. In order to chew, food must be between the teeth. For children who have difficulty moving food within the mouth, it may be placed by the parent or therapist to one side between the teeth. Experience will show if a child chews better on one side of the mouth than the other.
6. Eating in front of a mirror will allow the child to check if his lips are closed and to monitor his chewing pattern (see Figure 6.8).
7. Stability of plates and dishes may be attained by the use of non-slip mats and suction bases. A dish with one vertical side against which food may be loaded on to the spoon or fork is helpful. A dish with a hollow base which is filled with hot water will keep food warm for the slow eater. The added weight will also help to stabilise the dish (see Figure 6.9).

Figure 6.8: Using a mirror to check lip closure whilst chewing

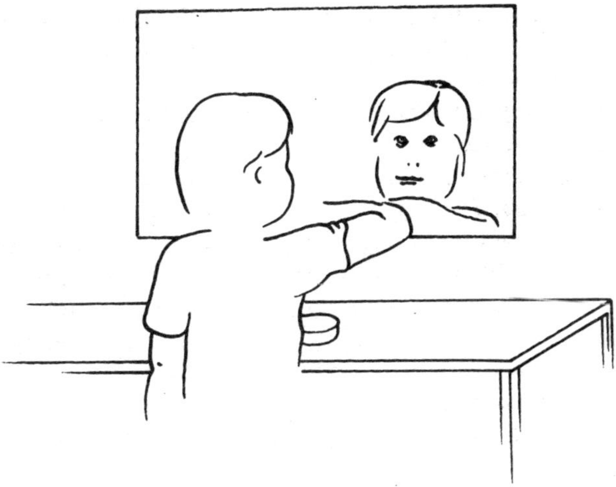

Figure 6.9: Dish with a hollow base which may be filled with hot water. Top view and side view of a dish with a vertical side against which food may be loaded on to a spoon or fork

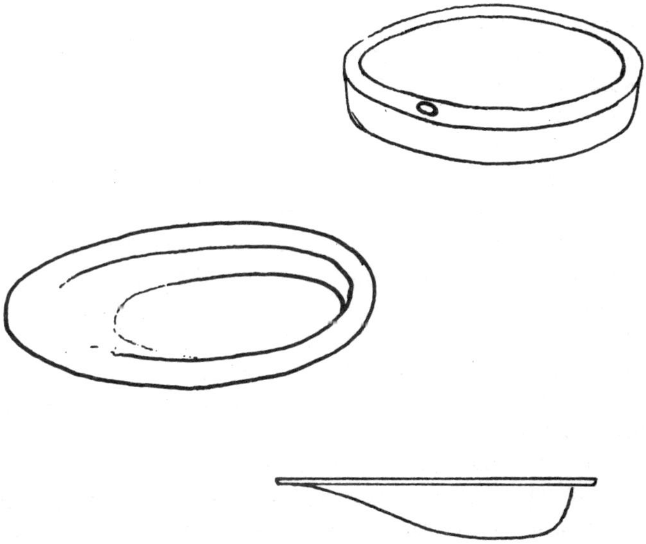

Figure 6.10: Assisted feeding using a long-handled spoon

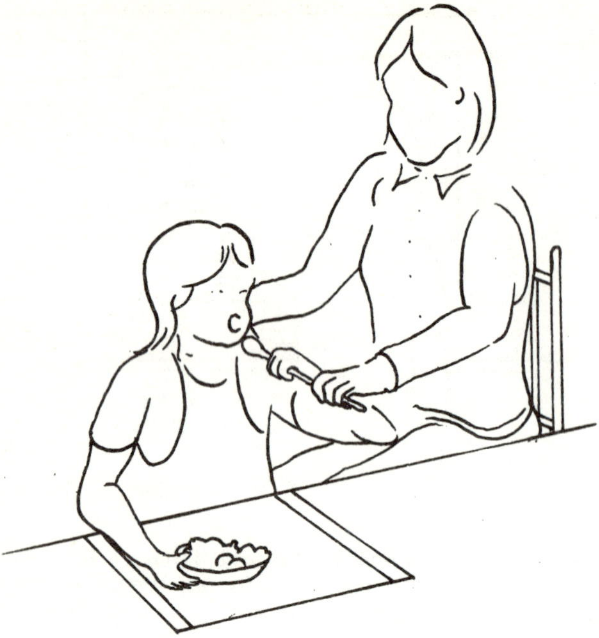

8. It may be possible to find cutlery which suits the needs of a particular child for one of the commercially available ranges.

   (a) Should the child have a strong bite reflex it will be more appropriate to select items made from shatter-proof plastic material or horn which being softer and warmer than metal tend not to stimulate this undesirable reflex so strongly.

   (b) Children who lack muscle power will feed themselves more effectively with lightweight cutlery so that implements when loaded with food will not be too heavy to manipulate.

9. The size of cutlery will depend upon the needs of the child. A long handle will facilitate assisted feeding (see Figure 6.10). A shallow spoon bowl will enable the child to take the food from it while it is in his mouth more easily than from a deep bowl.

10. A foam or commercially available handle will enable some children to grip more easily. Other children will benefit from a strap attached to each end of the handle through which their hand is placed so that the spoon or fork is not dropped whenever an adequate grip of it is not maintained (see Figure 6.11).

Figure 6.11: Spoon with foam rubber grip which enlarges the handle and increases friction thus making it easier to hold. Spoon with strap so that the child with poor grip does not drop it. Spoons with bowls bent in various ways to suit the needs of particular children

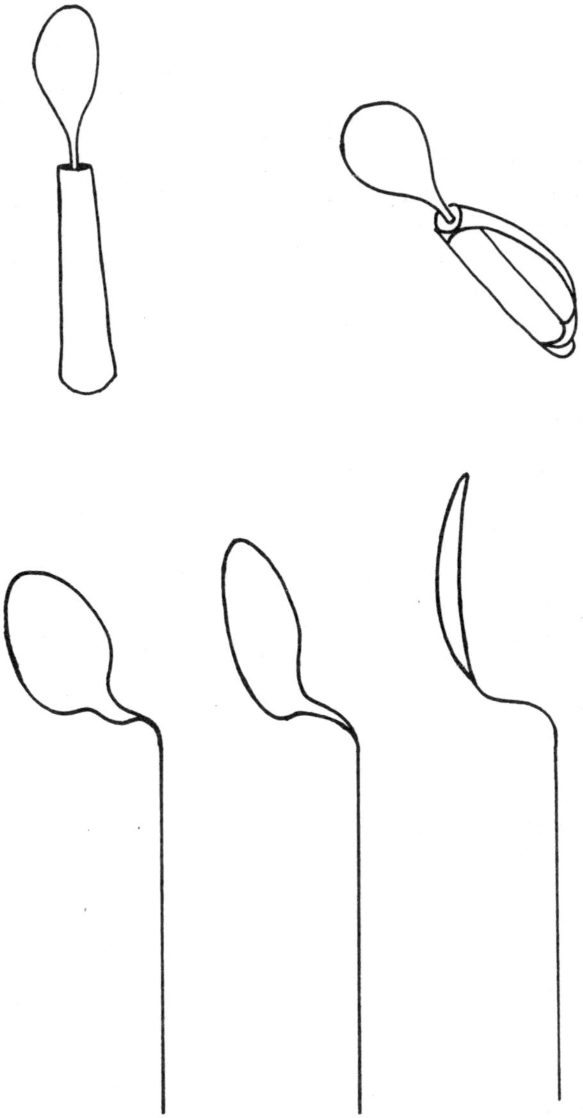

11. It may be necessary to bend or twist the handles of cutlery from some children so that they may reach their mouth with it. These adaptations are often very successful despite the alteration in trajectory being made both to suit the loading of the spoon or fork with food from the plate and the depositing of food in the mouth (see Figure 6.11).

There are children who will require far more radical adaptations of crockery and cutlery in order to feed independently. Conditions such as arthrogryposis and limb deficiency often call for greater ingenuity on the part of the occupational therapist (Rockey and Nelham, 1984, pp. 352–3).

Whatever the child's problems with feeding he will spend only a small proportion of his mealtimes in a clinical situation; the vast majority of his meals will be eaten at home. It is vital that his parents are conversant with the therapeutic aims for their child and are able to put them into practice.

DRESSING

The age at which most children are able to dress themselves varies according to personality, interest in the activity and opportunity to practise doing it (Illingworth, 1980, p. 140). It will also vary according to the child's manual dexterity and his perception of his own position in space and spatial relationships, among other skills. By the age of four most children are able to dress themselves except for difficult buttons and laces.

There are times when most children are reluctant to dress. The child who will *never* dress himself, even with suitable clothes, is very likely to have some difficulty which is preventing him from doing so. Should the task require an unusually large amount of concentration and effort the child may be reluctant even to attempt independent dressing. Such children often have general difficulties with co-ordination, a degree of dyspraxia and/or perceptual difficulties which give the overall impression of clumsiness. Difficulty with dressing may be the first indication the lay person has of the child's problems.

Other children have more obvious difficulties of a neurological, muscular or articulatory nature from which difficulties with dressing may be foreseen. For such children independent dressing may always be difficult and require specially adapted clothing and self-help adaptations to put them on.

Figure 6.12: Using a hoop to learn the concept of 'over the head'

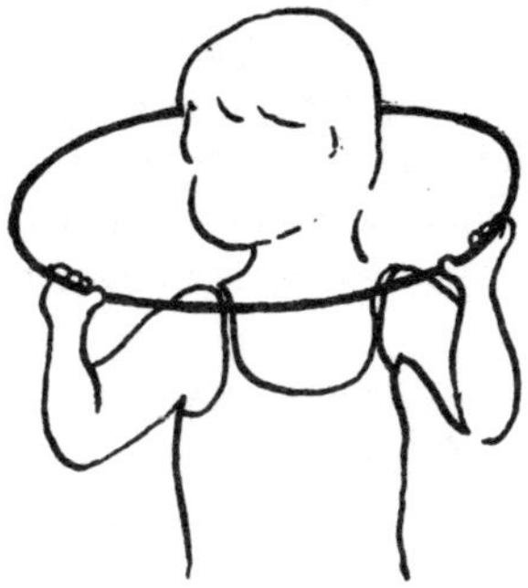

Helping the child to undress and dress

1. For the child who has severe motor or perceptual difficulties a predressing programme may be appropriate.
   (a) A large plastic hoop or a quoit can be used to teach the concept and movements of 'over the head', 'up an arm', 'up a leg' (see Figure 6.12).
   (b) Later a piece of material with a large hole cut out of the middle may be used in the same way so that the child learns to handle unstructured materials.
   (c) A full length mirror is useful for the child to monitor his movements with hoops, the material with a large hole in it and dressing-up cloths.
2. As with other skills the first need is for stability, usually in sitting, though many children eventually find their own optimum position for putting on and removing particular garments.
3. As children usually learn to undress before they learn to dress they should be taught in this order.
4. Loose-fitting clothes, particularly those with raglan armholes are easier to manage. Encourage parents to buy clothes for their child which are a *little* on the large side.
5. There is more elasticity in knitted fabrics than woven ones. Natural fibres are advisable, they slip more easily over the skin than synthetic ones, they absorb perspiration without feeling damp and have better insulating properties. These properties add greatly to the comfort of the child who cannot adjust his position independently

and are important for children who have poor circulation such as those suffering from spina bifida.

6. All occupational therapists are conversant with adapting garments to suit individual needs by enlarging openings and simplifying fastenings and by substituting Velcro for difficult buttons and press fasteners. Simple devices such as loops on underpants will aid pulling up for children with a variety of conditions including JCA, hemiplegia and other conditions where power and joint movement is limited.

7. Self-help adaptations should be kept as simple and as few as possible: a dressing stick with a hook at one end and non-slip handle rubber at the other is probably the most useful.

8. Children who are of a non-standard shape or size may require clothes specially designed and made. This can be an expensive problem for parents unless one of them, or an obliging relative or friend, is proficient with a sewing machine. Children for whom it is impossible to buy standard sized clothing may be helped by having a basic pattern block made to their individual measurements from which a variety of garments may be made. This ploy is particularly helpful for children of very small stature often with a disproportionately large head which may be caused by conditions such as achondroplasia or Morquio's syndrome. As these children grow older it is usually impossible to buy clothes to fit their small stature which are sufficiently sophisticated for their years. In the teenage years, fashionable clothes are important for self-esteem and fashion changes at an extraordinarily rapid rate!

Detailed accounts of dressing and clothing for children who suffer from cerebral palsy may be found in *Helping the Cerebral Palsied Children at Home* by Nancie H. Finnie and for children suffering from muscular dystrophy and allied neuromuscular diseases in *With a Little Help, Volume 2* by Philippa Harpin.

7

Motor Skills and Formal Education

The direction in which education starts a man, will determine his future life.

Plato, The Republic (4th Century, BC)

In the Western world education usually refers to learning in a formal setting, i.e. school. All children are required to attend school for a certain number of years, including children who suffer from one or a number of impairments. Some of the latter will be educated in school alongside their able peers and others will attend schools which provide special facilities to fill their needs. The needs of the child must be very carefully weighed against each other before decisions are made regarding school placement.

AREAS OF CONSIDERATION

There are three main areas which must be considered when making educational plans all of which concern the occupational therapist: the child; the school; the attitudes towards the child's impairments.

The child and his limitations

The needs of the child must be assessed against the background of his abilities and impairments. His motor skills must be assessed at both a gross and fine level. Is he, for instance, independently mobile or does he require special equipment such as a walking frame or a wheelchair at all times? Has he normal ability to learn but difficulty in recording on paper or verbally expressing his knowledge?

Careful planning during the pre-school years and continuing consultation with the child's teachers will reduce the number of disabilities from which he will suffer during his schooldays and may reduce the number of situations in which he is handicapped. For example, impairment of fine motor ability may preclude the use of a pen or pencil on paper but it does not prevent the child from recording by effective methods, such as an electric typewriter, computer or dictaphone. The impairment need not be a disability.

The school building

If the child has limited independent mobility, is confined to a wheelchair or has opted to use a mechanical means of mobility, access to the school will be important. Uneven paths leading to the building may make the passage of a wheelchair difficult. Steps at the entrance will require ramps located in such positions that they are not a hazard to able children entering the building. Changes in level between different parts of a classroom or between classrooms and passageways will, of course, limit the freedom of the child confined to a wheelchair. A school built on more than one storey will require the addition of a lift to make all parts accessible to the child in the wheelchair.

Some children need special toilet facilities in order to be independent; others will require the help of an adult acquainted with their needs. These special needs, even though they take up only a minute proportion of the school day, can ultimately be the ones on which decisions will be made about the school that a child will attend. Will help with toileting involve the child's mother attending him several times a day or will the education authority need to employ ancillary staff to help him. It is often the occupational therapist who is able to help the child attain the necessary degree of independence or suggest ways in which simple adaptations may be made to toilet facilities.

Attitudes towards the child's impairments

This will include the child's attitude towards himself, his self-esteem, his motivation to succeed and his attitude towards his peers. The child's attitudes will have been influenced from birth by his parents and other members of the family. The child who has been encouraged to mix with and play alongside other children and who has not been over-protected because of his impairments is more likely to settle successfully and profitably into school. The child whose family have realistic aspirations for him is likely to have the necessary self-image to make relationships with his peers. These are points which the occupational therapist should consider throughout all her contacts with the child and his family because attitudes develop gradually over the years and once formed are difficult to alter.

For the child who will attend a school which is predominantly for able pupils the attitudes of the staff must also be considered. Teachers who are unfamiliar with particular impairments may be apprehensive about having such a child in their class. Teachers can often be helped to adopt a more realistic attitude towards the problems of a particular child if they understand more about the condition: what the child can accomplish independently, in what situations he will need assistance and which tasks he will not be able to perform. It is not always possible to provide clear-cut answers to many questions for the demands made on the child and his abilities are likely to change as he progresses through school. Time should be spent answering queries, explaining the nature of a child's difficulties and assuring the teacher that further visits will be made by the occupational therapist, or at least that she will be available on the telephone to discuss and perhaps suggest solutions to problems which may arise in the future.

Seating and positioning

This may be one of the first problems to be faced when a child begins school. The problem may be the position in which the child should sit or be supported in to be able to see and hear the activities in the classroom, and to perform fine motor activities. He may need a chair and table of different dimensions because of his small stature. It should be decided whether the child should be seated in his optimal working position or be fully integrated into his peer group. Will he need to sit in his wheelchair all day with a suitable table or tray on which to work? Will he be able to transfer himself to a more conventional chair? Will he need help every time he does so and will he need to be lifted into each new position?

Special equipment

The child may need special apparatus if he is to perform at his optimum level. If the child uses a typewriter or computer with a printer to produce written work, he will need to keep his work in

Figure 7.1: Self-opening scissors, palmar grip scissors and whole-hand grip self-opening scissors

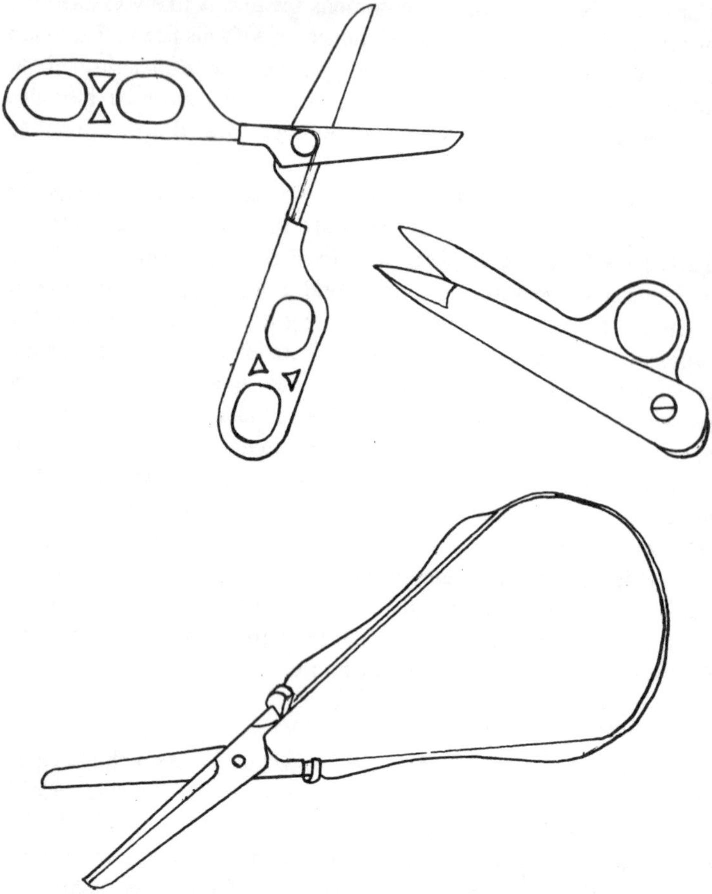

a looseleaf file rather than an exercise book. Small differences such as this are better discussed before the child enters school for many teachers find them difficult to cope with during their full day.

Can the child turn over the pages of a book easily? The child with severe difficulties may need a page turner, a cantilevered non-slip blade and handle or even an electric page turner. For the child with only slight difficulty, slipping a paper clip on to the side of each page will separate them sufficiently for him to turn them.

Conventional scissors require finger movements; whole hand grip, self-opening scissors require only a whole hand squeezing movement. The simple operation of these scissors allows children who cannot use ordinary scissors to take part in cutting activities. These scissors are also available attached to a block so that only one extended downward hand movement is required for cutting (see Figure 7.1).

Minor motor difficulties

A child's minor motor difficulties may pass unnoticed by his teachers during his first year or so in school. Often physical education is conducted on a very informal basis without instruction to perform precise movements. In this situation the child will move as he feels confident to do and his lack of co-ordination may pass unnoticed. Similarly when the child is asked to copy his name or a short sentence describing a picture he has drawn, poor motor control may not be obvious. It will only be when larger amounts of written work are expected and the child is required not only to form letters but also to compose sentences, sequence stories and recall how to spell the words therein that the problem may become apparent.

If an occupational therapist has known and has assessed the child for some time before he reaches school age she will have foreseen these difficulties and will have initiated a remedial programme to develop the child's motor skills to their optimum level and provide self-help adaptations.

Suggestions to help fine motor development

1. Encourage leading with the index finger with toys which are operated by pressing a small button, for example Jack-in-a-box, toy cash register, dialling on a telephone and finger painting.
2. Encourage precise index finger/thumb grip:
   (a) picking up hundreds and thousands which have been thinly scattered;
   (b) picking up and placing small pegs in a pegboard;
   (c) pegging clothes on a washing line with spring pegs;
   (d) action singing games which include index finger/thumb opposition.
3. Encourage specific fine hand movements:
   (a) finger painting;
   (b) drawing with a finger dipped in water on a chalkboard;

(c) running a finger along the lines of grouting between the tiles in the bathroom;
(d) drawing with a finger on steamy windows.

4. Encourage drawing ability according to the child's developmental level.
The abilities of the average child are as follows:

2 years:	imitates a vertical stroke
2.5 years:	imitates a horizontal stroke
3 years:	copies a circle, imitates a cross
4 years:	copies a cross and a square
5 years:	copies a triangle
Between 6 and 7 years:	copies a diamond

Devise games which give a child guidance to draw in the desired direction.
(a) Draw a vertical or horizontal road and a car at the start of it. Ask the child to draw a line along the road in the direction in which the car will travel.
(b) Draw a line of flower heads. Ask the child to provide the vertical flower stems.
(c) Ask the child to draw a geometric shape by drawing inside the appropriate stencil (see Figure 7.2). He should use the stencil a number of times so that he learns the required movement. Encourage him to continue by making the shapes he has drawn into objects, e.g. a square can become a window, a house or a garden; a triangle can become a tepee or a road traffic sign. With continued practice the child will learn the movements required to make the shape and be able to draw them free hand.

5. For the child who is reluctant to attempt to draw a human figure, first draw it for him talking through the parts as they appear and relating them to the child's own body. Draw a circular shape for a face, add one eye and encourage the child to add the other one. Draw a mouth and encourage the child to add to it. Draw hair and encourage the child to add more. Accept his efforts, do not criticise them or suggest improvements.

6. Use a floor chalkboard and chalk especially if the child lacks stability or has a tremor because
(a) kneeling on the floor is a more stable position than sitting on a chair;
(b) both the chalkboard and chalk have matt surfaces and therefore provide more friction than pencil or crayon on paper;

Figure 7.2: Drawing inside stencils teaches the child the movements required to draw geometric shapes

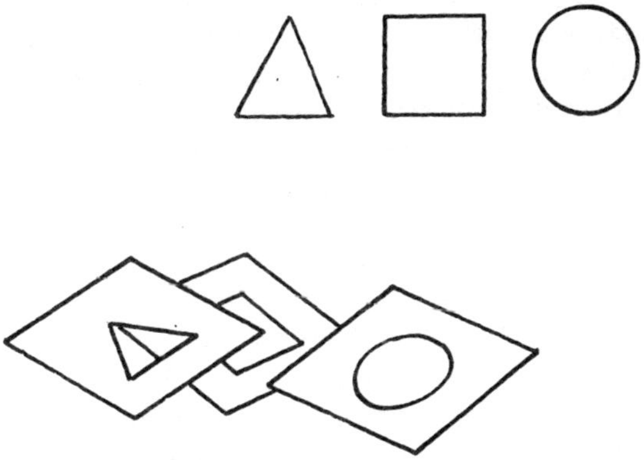

(c) a mark made on paper is permanent, those made on a chalkboard may be instantly erased. This prevents visual reinforcement of errors. The child who is afraid that he will make mistakes should be given a duster so that he may erase his efforts which do not satisfy him.

The occupational therapist will have explained to the child's parents the difficulties he may experience as larger amounts of written work are required in school and the alternative methods which are available to overcome them, should it prove to be necessary. In the same way the teacher's doubts about a child's ability to cope with large amounts of written work at speed may be dispelled.

Schools vary in the amount of instruction which it is thought desirable to give children who are just beginning to write. Some allow children to copy letters in whatever fashion they are able while others insist on the correct manner of letter formation being taught from the beginning. For the majority of children it is immaterial which method is used; eventually they will learn to write in an acceptable manner. A minority of children, particularly those with dyspraxic-type difficulties, will be unable to write unless they are shown exactly *how* to form the letters. Showing the child each movement entailed in the formation of each letter, reinforced by a verbal commentary is often successful, particularly if similarly formed letters are studied in groups.

Some children are first referred because they have writing

difficulties after having been in school for some time. It is important to ascertain that their basic difficulty is with writing because often it is only a symptom of a wider range of difficulties which may include problems at both a gross and fine motor level. Until a child begins school he has often been given little direction to his activities. He will naturally have chosen the activities with which he has met with success and thus his problems have passed unnoticed. In addition, because of avoidance, he will have had less practice than the average child with fine motor skills.

Case note

Mark was referred for occupational therapy at the age of seven because of severe handwriting difficulties. He had made good progress with reading, spelling and number work. Full assessment revealed that he had severe dyspraxia which affected both gross and fine motor skills and the use of language. The latter caused him to be a figure of fun in the classroom for frequently he could not produce the appropriate word. On one occasion when asked to name a picture of a swan and was unable to find the word 'swan', he described it as 'a ducky swimmer with feathers'.

Occupational therapy proceeded with activities to improve his gross motor performance but Mark only learned movements which were very painstakingly taught, there was no carry over into other activities because he did not have the ability to plan spontaneous movement. At a fine level he seemed to be incapable of retaining the necessary patterns of movement to improve his handwriting. A programme of learning the keyboard of an electric typewriter was started and with weekly lessons, Mark attained a speed of 15 words a minute. He used his typewriter for written work in school and was able to produce written work commensurate with his peers.

His parents described him as a child who had never enjoyed outdoor play, who had no interest in learning to ride a bicycle. Indoors he had learned to operate a cassette recorder and record player at an early age. He loved watching television, especially horse racing, and had gained prestige within his extended family by being able to remember the form of race horses and quickly working out the betting odds. In this manner Mark had diverted attention from his severe dyspraxia until he entered junior school.

On other occasions a referral because of handwriting difficulties may lead to the discovery of other difficulties connected with the written word. A piece of creative writing has a number of elements

— the sequence of the piece as a whole, the construction of sentences, the choice of words and the ability to spell those words. Children who have difficulty with any of these elements often spend time thinking about what to write and how to spell, all the time their pencil dithering over the paper; the work that results appears to demonstrate handwriting difficulties when the basic problem is with language. Questioning parents often reveals that these children have had early language problems which may have required speech therapy. Careful assessment will reveal the precise nature of the difficulties which may indicate that further help is required from a speech therapist, an educational psychologist and an occupational therapist.

Case note

Graham had attended a child development centre since he was a few weeks old because he suffered from spina bifida. During his first years therapy was concerned with attaining balance and stability in sitting and preventing spinal and hip deformity. From three to five years he attended a weekly group for children suffering from spina bifida which concentrated on teaching social skills and the perception of self and space through games and action songs.

At five years he began his formal education at his local primary school, his occupational therapist liaising with his teachers regarding mobility in his wheelchair and the precautions necessary because of the lack of sensation in his lower limbs. His education psychologist assessed his IQ to be exactly average and there was no significant discrepancies in his scores in subtests.

At the age of eight he was again referred for occupational therapy because of handwriting difficulties. Assessment showed that he adopted a good overall position for writing and that he had a dynamic tripod pencil grip. He formed letters in the correct manner and had no difficulty with spacing between words. The nature of his difficulty was revealed when he was asked to write a short creative piece; his problems included constructing sentences and sequencing his ideas. As he pondered over the contents of the piece, his pencil dithered over the paper, sometimes making unintentional marks on it. The time he spent in thought gave the impression that he was an extremely slow writer. The supposed handwriting difficulty was, in fact, a language problem.

Helping the child with handwriting difficulties

1. The first consideration is the child's overall sitting position. His table and chair should be of a suitable height for him and in relation to one another. It is preferable that his paper rests on a surface which slopes slightly towards him. When children begin to write they usually do so on a single sheet of paper. Writing will be more comfortable if the surface on which it rests is covered with heavy sugar (construction) paper which will provide slight cushioning.

2. The *paper* should be of good quality so that it will not crease under the child's fist.

(a) Most children cope best with paper which has a matt surface because it provides more friction and thus better control of the writing tool. A few children who have difficulty with smooth movements or who have very poor muscle power benefit from using paper with a slightly glossy surface.

(b) Children who are beginning to write are usually given A5 (148 x 21 mm) paper. It is best if the child writes along the longer side of the paper so that the page contains only a few lines of writing and he will not need to adjust its position or change his writing position as he progressed down the page.

(c) The child who is just beginning to write letters most usually uses unlined paper. Children differ in the time when they are able to use lined paper and in the width of line which is best for them. Some children find paper with four lines helpful and which indicates the height of small letters such as *a*, *e*, *o*, and the position of ascenders and descenders (see Figure 7.3). The needs of each individual child should be considered when choosing paper for him, his chronological age and the paper suited to his peers do not necessarily dictate his needs.

3. *Pencils* and *pens* too should be chosen to suit the needs of each individual child.

(a) The thickness of pens and pencils should suit the needs of the child. It does not necessarily follow that very young children manage best with thick pencils and crayons. A writing implement of small diameter requires a finer grip than a thicker one. Some children find the former easier to control. Thicker ones do not require such close opposition of the fingers and thumb.

(b) A heavy writing implement increases resistance to gravity which helps to decrease tremor for some children (see Figure 7.4).

(c) The type of tool a child uses for drawing and writing should

Figure 7.3: Paper with four lines which helps the child to gauge the relative sizes and positions of letters

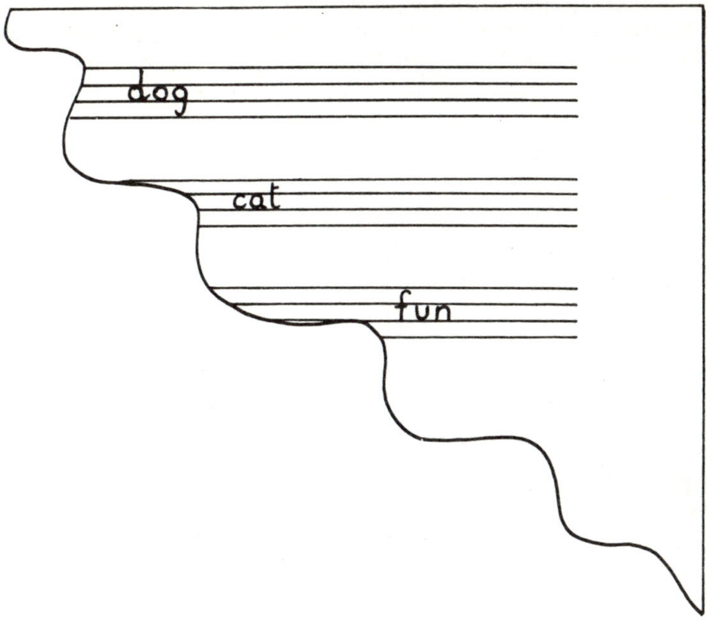

not depend on his age but on his needs. It is, for example, customary for children of infant school age to use a pencil and for pens to be introduced at about eight or nine years of age. Some young children benefit from using felt-tipped and fibre-tipped pens rather than crayons and pencils because more friction is provided by the former.

(d) For the child who can use only a whole hand horizontal grip a T-bar may be fitted to a short pencil or crayon (see Figure 7.4).

(e) Only rarely are ball-point pens suitable for writing. Because the writing tip is a ball-bearing it provides no friction and it is therefore difficult to control.

4. The *grip* with which the writing tool is held will affect the quality of drawing and writing. The adoption of a tripod grip usually begins at about two and a half years. At the age of seven, children begin to adopt a dynamic tripod grip (Ziviani, 1982).

(a) The precise nature of the grip will depend on the dimension of the child's hand. For example, it will be impossible for the

Figure 7.4: A pencil with added weight at the end which helps to reduce some tremors. A pencil with a triangular grip to encourage a dynamic tripod and to indicate the place on the shaft where the pencil should be held. Two crayons taped together in a T-shape for the child who can only use a horizontal whole hand grip

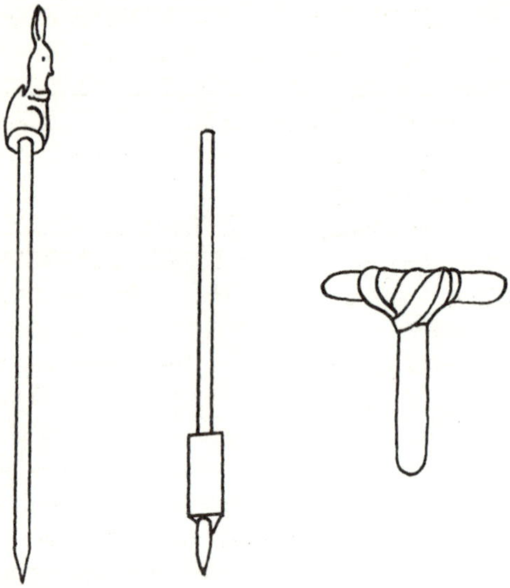

child with particularly long digits to hold the writing tool with the pads of the thumb and index finger level without flexion of the index finger at the proximal joint.

(b) The angle to the vertical at which the child holds his writing tool will depend on the nature of that tool. For example, a ball-point pen must be held almost vertically so that the ball bearing tip is in contact with the paper.

(c) Some children hold a writing tool with the fingers almost on the tip, perhaps in an unconscious attempt to attain better control of it. Others hold it high up the shaft which provides inadequate control of fine movement. It may be possible to make use of grip marks which are an integral part of the tool to guide the child as to where he should hold it. A triangular grip fitted to the tool at the appropriate point will also give guidance to the correct gripping point (see Figure 7.4).

(d) A dynamic tripod grip, where movement is isolated to the fingers, is necessary for flowing writing. A triangular pencil grip helps to develop such a grip providing a side on which to rest the thumb, another for the index finger, the third side indicating the position of the middle finger (see Figure 7.4).

(e) Many children learn to use a dynamic tripod spontaneously; others after its importance has been explained to them and practice provided. Because of motor difficulties some children find a tripod grip ineffective. A tremor or lack of muscle power may lead a child to adopt a grip with the index, middle and ring fingers spread down the shaft of the writing tool. Others will flex their fingers at both interphalangeal joints with the thumb across the shaft of the writing tool. For such children it may not be possible to attain a dynamic tripod.

(f) It has been suggested that left-handed people are more likely than right-handers to adopt a hooked (inverted) hand while writing. However, a hooked hand has been observed in both left- and right-handed people and research has shown that the adoption of a hooked hand posture indicates that the subject has the dominant cerebral hemisphere on the same side as the preferred writing hand; it is more usual for the preferred hand and cerebral dominance to be on opposite sides (Levy and Reid, 1976). Personal observation suggests that a hooked hand while writing is concerned not only with hand posture but also with cerebral organisation. Care should be taken, therefore, before attempting to change the degree of flexion in which a child holds his hand whilst writing.

5. Many children learn correct *letter formation* with a normal amount of instruction. Others, particularly those who have difficulty with motor organisation, will have difficulty learning correct letter formation.

(a) Demonstrate to the child the exact movements he should make. Let him copy the appropriate movement as it is being made.

(b) Mark where to begin describing each character and if necessary add an arrow to indicate the direction in which the child should proceed.

(c) The child should understand that the formation of all letters except *d* and *e*, and all numbers should start at the top.

(d) Teach the letters in groups. For example, if the child is taught lower case *c* he has already learned the beginning of *a*, *o*, *d*, *q* and *g*. Teach letters with a bridge or inverted bridge shape as a group, i.e. *m*, *n*, *h*, *u*, *w* and *y* (Alston and Taylor, 1984).

(e) It is advisable to check with the child's teacher the precise style of writing used in his school. Children who have difficulty with letter construction are often unable to cope with slight differences in the style of letters.

Alternative methods of recording information

1. *Electric typewriters*, office and portable models. Electric models are preferable to manual ones because the quality of type produced on the paper does not depend on how the keys are struck. Children who need to use a typewriter rarely have the necessary sharp finger movements to produce consistent typing with a manual machine. Large office models are stronger than the portable type which are intended for occasional home use. The so-called portable models are not suitable for the child to carry from classroom to classroom; many of them weigh about 11 kg.
2. *Electronic printers* are easily portable machines, some weighing as little as 2 kg. They fit easily on to a standard school table or desk, the smallest being the dimensions of A4 size paper. Models may be either mains or battery powered, the latter allowing the child more choice with seating as he does not need to be near a power point. Many models are almost soundless. Some have an illuminated display of the last 15 to 20 keys which have been struck enabling the child to check his work and correct it if necessary before it is printed. This last feature may be confusing for some children as the last character displayed will appear on the right and the whole display will move towards the left. Because of the predetermined size of the display area, half a word may appear at the beginning of it which may confuse some children. Some machines can prove expensive to run because they require special thermal paper or a single strike ribbon. For children at secondary school, college and university students these disadvantages may be outweighed by the machine's portability and silent operation.
3. *Microcomputers* with a VDU, word processing program and printer can provide a suitable means of recording in schools. Many homes now possess a microcomputer which with word processing capabilities and a printer will provide a suitable way of doing homework and other writing. The advantages are that the child, after learning the word processing system, will be able to see a large display of his writing, before it is printed, which can be corrected until he is satisfied with his efforts. Whenever possible, a printer which produces solid print should be used, especially if the child has

any visual difficulties. Dot matrix heads print more quickly than daisywheels but this will seldom be a consideration with the relatively small amount of work produced by a school child. The newer dot matrix printers produce print of 'near letter quality' but even this is not quite solid; because of the printing method there are no true descenders on letter characters which can confuse children who have form constancy problems or difficulty with the relative sizes of letters when they write with a pen.

4. There is other equipment available for children with more serious hand difficulties.

(a) Keyguards which help to guide the finger down to the appropriate key.

(b) Continuous rolls of paper for those unable to insert paper in a machine. The child leaves appropriate spaces between pieces of work which may later be separated by the teacher or parent.

(c) A forearm support will help the child who lacks muscle power and will reduce the effects of a tremor for some children.

(d) An expanded keyboard will enable the child with only crude manual control to type.

(e) Mini keyboards are available for children with limited hand movement. Machines such as the Microwriter which has only six keys, combinations of which produce all the functions of a normal keyboard, will enable some children with only some finger movement to type. It has an illuminated display or it may be connected to a VDU when a larger display will be seen. It is very portable, looks like a very 'normal' piece of equipment and has a memory which will store several pages of print.

(f) For the severely handicapped child, systems are available which are operated by means of joysticks, touchpads and suck-blow devices.

Children who will benefit from using a keyboard

1. Those who will never have sufficient fine motor control to use a pen or pencil.

2. Those who have poor fine motor skills and who will take much longer than the average child to learn to write legibly and quickly. Writing is much more than putting marks on paper since it also includes the skills of spelling, constructing sentences and sequencing information. The child who has difficulty learning to write and construct letters without conscious thought will not be free to

practise the other writing skills mentioned above. Removing the motor planning element from written work by the use of some form of keyboard will allow him to experience creative writing. Should his handwriting improve (which is often the case when an alternative method of recording is provided) he will of course use a pen, but his keyboard skills will be useful for computer work and in later life.

3. Older children who have mastered handwriting but lack the necessary speed when larger written output is required of them.

Teaching keyboard skills

1. Accurate positioning is required to ensure that the child can reach the keyboard while his elbows are in mid flexion and that he can also see the print on the paper which is over the platen, displayed on the VDU or the illuminated display.
2. The child should be taught to put two sheets of paper into the machine, one to type on, the other a backing sheet to prevent wear on the platen.
3. To ensure the paper is aligned with the rows of print, turn the platen or repeatedly press the carriage return key until 3 or 4 cm of paper is visible. Release the tension on the platen and pull the paper through, aligning the two top corners with the bottom two, return the lever to apply platen tension. Turn the paper down to the required position at the top of the page.
4. For the child who is unlikely to be able to manipulate a pencil effectively, begin teaching keyboard skills when the child would normally begin to use crayons. Provide him with outline drawings which he will 'colour' with the appropriate typed letter, e.g. a picture of a *t*eapot will be 'coloured' with *t*, a *d*uck with *d* (Goad, 1977). In this way a young child can enjoy 'scribbling' on paper and at the same time begin to learn the positions of letters on the keyboard (see Figure 7.5).
5. Children of school age who are beginning to learn to read and who would normally be beginning to write can learn the keyboard using exercises which have been simplified from a normal typing manual.
6. Set the typewriter at wide line spacing because young children need print widely spaced as in their first reading books. Set wide margins so that the lines of type will be, at the most, forty characters wide which compares with the number of letter characters and

Figure 7.5: Pictures for the young child to 'colour' with a typewriter using the appropriate letter character

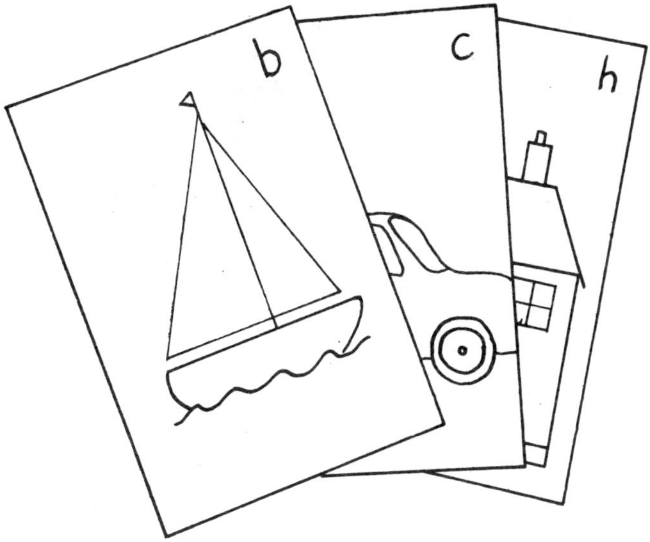

spaces a young child would handwrite along one line.
7. Use a vertical method of teaching the keyboard because the exercises will entail only one finger at a time so that it is possible to adjust the system according to the finger function of the child.
8. Prepare each exercise on a separate card. Colour code the cards so that all those for the left hand have a red mark on them, for example, and those for the right hand have a green mark. For some children it is helpful to put a similar mark on the typewriter keys to remind the child which hand he is to use. It is also useful for some children to have a small mark on the back of each of their hands so that typing cards, typewriter and their hands are co-ordinated. For the child who has difficulty with form constancy it may be necessary to cover the upper case letters on the keys with lower case ones.
9. On each card denote which hand and finger the child should use and what exactly he should type including the spaces. It is often beneficial to train the child to type two spaces after each word or element of a typing exercise. Underneath these instructions, prepare a small example of how the completed exercise should look (see Figure 7.6).
10. Aim for a smooth regular typing action in the first instance,

Figure 7.6: Typing exercises — each on a separate card which is colour coded according to the hand to be used. Each card denotes the finger and hand to be used, exactly what the child should type and an example of the completed exercise

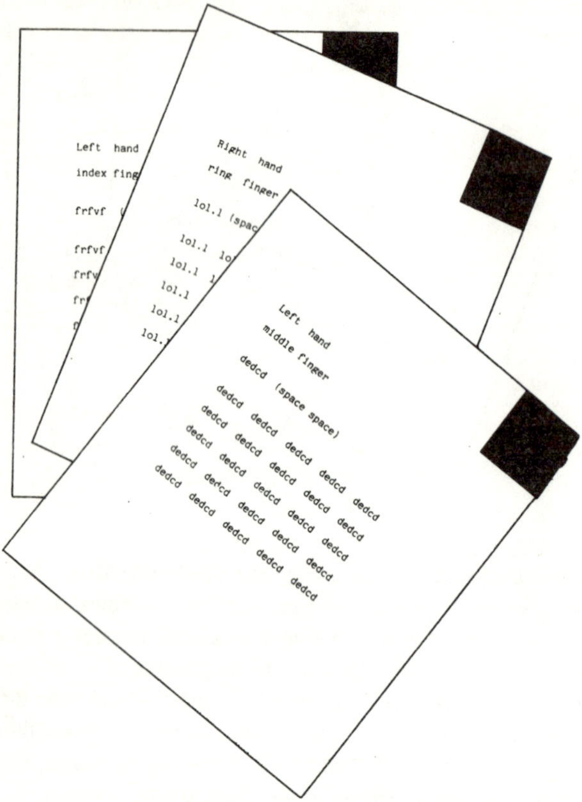

speed will follow later. At first the therapist and the child should name each letter as it is typed, later the child alone may do so. It is very important that the child says and thinks about each letter as it is typed otherwise he will not learn the keyboard but only be practising a series of movements.

11. Whenever possible teach the child always to use his right thumb for the space bar. Some children, of course, will be unable to use their right thumb or perhaps other digits; some will only have the use of one hand. Using a vertical method of teaching the keyboard will allow the occupational therapist to adapt the programme accordingly.

12. When the child has learned part of the keyboard he will be able to write words, where possible using both hands. This is an essential part of the programme because it allows the child to see that his practice is already providing him with realistic skills.
13. As the child has practised his typing exercises he will have learned the function of the return key. Next teach him how to use the shift key for capital letters, depressing the shift key on the opposite side of the machine to where the letter is being typed.
14. The next step is copy typing. Pieces of appropriate length should be prepared on separate cards, using short lines and wide line spacing.
15. The final step is being able to type original work. When children begin to write their teacher often writes what they wish to say and the child copies it. This method is also useful for the child who uses a typewriter. Another step towards independent creative typing is to prepare work cards with sentences with one word omitted which the child must insert, e.g. My name is ______; I like ______; My birthday is on ______.
16. For any typist the transition from copy typing to creative typing is a big step which requires a great deal of practice. Allow the child plenty of time to establish this skill.
17. Children attending schools with special facilities for physical disabilities will probably have provision made in their curriculum for learning keyboard skills. Those who need to type but attend a primary school which has only a few pupils with special needs will benefit from being taught these skills before their machine is introduced into the classroom; unfortunately few teachers have the necessary time available to teach one child these special skills.

8

Subjective and Objective Observation of the Child

I keep six honest serving-men
(They taught me all I know);
Their names are What and Why and When
And How and Where and Who.

Rudyard Kipling

As we have seen, impairment concerns the whole child and involves all those who come into contact with him. For the child to work towards the prevention of impairment becoming disability or handicap and for his family, teachers and therapists to facilitate this, his abilities and problems must be defined and strategies evolved to allow him to live a life of maximum opportunity to learn and develop his potential. Ideally this process will be a continuous one: problems being defined against the background of the child's developmental level, suitable strategies being devised by which the child may actively work towards the defined goal reassessment in order to define future goals, and so on.

For every child there is the first meeting with the occupational therapist where she may be alone or with some of the other therapists and medical staff who will become involved with him. The child may be a a young baby, a toddler, a junior school child or an adolescent thinking ahead to the time he leaves school and the degree of independence he may hope to achieve. There are basic principles which may be applied to children of all ages and to almost any type of impairment. Within these principles the various observation, assessment and treatment techniques will be reduced or augmented to the child's condition, his needs and those of his family.

Background information

Before meeting the child and his family, it is advisable to take a brief look at any medical notes. The child may have undergone previous detailed assessment and it would be futile to repeat every detail of it. Previous notes will provide information which the therapist needs prior to assessment and treatment. The parents may have been questioned a number of times about their child's history; consulting the hospital notes removes the need to repeat this irksome procedure yet again. It also helps to create a good early relationship if the occupational therapist is aware of the basic details regarding the child. Care should be taken, however, not to let the current assessment be coloured by the opinions of others. Basic facts should be assimilated but conclusions should be drawn only from current subjective and objective observations.

Social information

It is important also to ascertain the social facts about the family before the first meeting. John Smith's mother may not be known as Mrs Smith, she may have remarried or never have been married at all. The adult male accompanying them may not be the father of the child or the mother's husband. The child may have been adopted so that details about the perinatal period may not be known. Parents may not wish to discuss such details as the child may not have been made aware that he is adopted. There are innumerable family situations with which parents would prefer not to be confronted particularly during an initial interview. Where the family situation seems unusual or is particularly complex discussion with the social worker, if there is one, will be particularly helpful. Embarrassment may be avoided by becoming familiar with the relationships within the family before the initial interview. Evaluation of the child's needs will be made more realistically if the physical and personal family situation is understood.

It is a comparatively simple matter for the occupational therapist to become conversant with the child and the family she is about to meet. The child and his family are not in the same position. A brief introduction of oneself together with a brief description of the assessment which is to follow helps to put both parents and their child at ease; it helps to remove apprehension about the unknown.

Overall plans to help the child and his family will be made

following a detailed assessment, estimate or evaluation of the child's potential which will be based on his observed and reported strengths and weaknesses. His observed behaviour will consist of what the occupational therapist sees and hears while they are together. His reported behaviour will be the subjective comments of the child, if he is able to express himself verbally, his parents, teachers and other people who care for him.

SUBJECTIVE INFORMATION

Parents have the most intimate knowledge of their child. They are with him night and day, when he is sick, when he is well, they help him to succeed and console him when he fails; they are with him when he is happy and when he is upset. Parents' observations regarding their child are a crucial part of any assessment procedure. Their observations should always be investigated even if previous assessments suggest they are unfounded. Theirs is not a professional view but the perceptive therapist will be able to make pertinent deductions from their reports of their child's behaviour.

Many centres which assess and treat children with chronic impairment produce their own questionnaire for parents and other carers. These questionnaires usually contain detailed questions about every aspect of the child's life: how he sleeps, how he is positioned during the day, the types of food he eats, what he drinks and how he takes them or is helped to do so, dressing procedures, play activities, how he communicates his needs and desires, his particular likes and dislikes. Sections are usually arranged in developmental order.

It is important that parents are introduced gently to such questionnaires and that it is not thrust upon them immediately after they meet the therapist. It is advisable to begin working on any such document *with* the parents to give them some idea of what is expected of them. This procedure also allows the therapist to ascertain the parents' level of literacy. Some adults have a specific difficulty in reading anything which is set in a formal manner and the nervousness and tension created for many parents by hospital or clinic visits may exacerbate these difficulties. People who have not attained a level of literacy necessary for the practicalities of daily life are reluctant to admit their inability and will go to extraordinary lengths to conceal it; some adults as well as children suffer from dyslexia.

Responses to questionnaires should always be discussed with

parents so that they are able to see the significance of their child's difficulties and understand how they may be helped.

QUESTIONS TO ASK PARENTS AND CARE STAFF

According to the situation the occupational therapist may ask the parents or carers to fill in the questionnaire and discuss their answers with them or she may find it more appropriate to pose the questions verbally and fill in the answers herself. Where the occupational therapist works as part of a multi- or intradisciplinary team it would be more appropriate to formulate one questionnaire which would serve the needs of all disciplines. This removes the need to repeat the same questions a number of times and reduces the amount of paper work for each child. It is helpful to provide space on the questionnaire for more than one set of answers so that it may be repeated at appropriate intervals and thus provide a record of the child's progress.

Not all the questions will be appropriate to every child and in some clinical situations it may be appropriate to formulate several questionnaires to the physical and mental conditions which are encountered.

The items in italics within brackets are comments on the questions and are not part of the questionnaire.

QUESTIONNAIRE

Name ________
Date of birth ________
Hospital Number ________

Background information

1. Are there other children in the family? What are their names and ages?
(The answers to these questions provide the therapist with topics of conversation with the child. The answers also indicate other family responsibilities, for instance, will the parents need appointments at times that leave them free to collect siblings from school.)
2. Does your child attend: a toddler group; a playgroup; day

nursery; a baby minder; school. If so, please give the name and address. Will you be happy for me to visit the establishment to make suggestions which will help your child during his time there?
(*It is important that all those involved with the child have the same aims and are working towards the same goals.*)
3. Has your child ever been seen by an occupational therapist before? Please give details. Is your child currently seeing another occupational therapist?
(*Occasionally, families are seen by both community and hospital based occupational therapists, each unaware of the other's involvement.*)
4. Is it difficult for you to make visits to this clinic? How long is your journey? Do you drive? Do you come on public transport? If you were asked to attend regularly would it be difficult to make arrangements for other children to be cared for? Would you need to take time off from work in order to attend?
(*The answers to these questions allow the therapist to make realistic plans for treatment programmes.*)

Movement

1. When your child is on the floor, how does he move? Does he roll? Does he push himself on his back? Does he creep or crawl? Does he drag himself along commando fashion? Does he shuffle on his bottom? Does he cruise holding on to furniture? Does he walk independently?
2. Does he fall more often than you would expect or more than your other children did? Where does he usually hurt himself when he falls?
(*A child who does not use saving reactions when falling — stretching out his arms and taking the fall on his hands — is likely to bump his nose or forehead.*)
Does he often trip over toys on the floor or frequently bump into furniture?
(*An affirmative answer suggests that vision and perception of spatial relationships should be investigated.*)
3. Can he negotiate stairs? Do you allow him to come down the stairs independently? Does he crawl up them? Does he walk up them holding onto the banisters? Does he also need to hold your hand? Does he walk up the stairs two feet to each step? Does he walk up in an adult fashion with alternate feet on each step? Is he able to

come down the stairs safely? Does he come down on his bottom? Does he slide down on his tummy? Does he walk down two feet to a step? Does he walk down with alternate feet on each step?
4. Is he confident when walking outside? Does he need a hand to hold? Is he able to walk on uneven ground such as an unmade up path or on grass? How far do you think he would walk without being overtired?
5. Does he have a tricycle or pedal car? Is he able to pedal it or does he paddle along with his feet on the ground? Does he have a bicycle? Is it fitted with stabilisers? Did he take longer than usual to learn to balance his bicycle? Is he able to steer the bicycle with one hand while he signals with the other? Does he find steering with one hand easier than with the other?
(*A particular difficulty with steering with one hand is often an indication of weakness in that hand or side*.)
Does he have any difficulty getting on or off the bicycle?
6. Does he ever go to a swimming pool? Does he enjoy being in the water? Is he able to swim? Which strokes does he prefer?
(*Many children who have co-ordination problems find breast stroke particularly difficult because both arm and leg movements are complex, each requiring concentrated effort. Children who have poor appreciation of their position in space are helped by visually monitoring their own movements. It is, of course, impossible to watch the legs moving during breast stroke*.)
Does he have any difficulty co-ordinating the movements of his arms and legs?

Chairs

1. Does your child use the same chairs as the rest of the family? Where does he usually sit? Does he seem comfortable and do you think it gives him the support he needs? Could you describe any special seating arrangements you have for your child? Who provided the seat? Have you made any adaptations to it, e.g. putting a cushion at the back or adding straps to keep him in position?
2. Does he find it difficult to sit in a chair? Does he fall to one side? Does he slip down out of it? Does he seem to stiffen and push back out of it? Does he need to support himself with his hands while sitting in some chairs?
3. Does he ride in a pushchair or wheelchair? What type is it? Are you happy with the chair or do you think he needs a different model?

Is the chair difficult to push? Is it easy to fold and put into your car? Can your child propel himself in his wheelchair? Does he tend to veer to one side when propelling himself? Have you brought it with you today?

Feeding

1. In what position does your child feed? Lying down? Sitting on your lap? On a special chair? With the rest of the family at the table?
2. Is he breast or bottle fed? Does he take solids? Are there any foods he does not like? Could you describe them?
3. Can he feed himself with a biscuit, bread or other foods which he can hold in his hands?
4. Does he attempt to feed himself with a spoon? Can he load the spoon himself? Can he carry the loaded spoon to his mouth? Can he close his lips round the spoon to take the food off it? Can he chew and swallow the food?
5. Can he manage a piece of cutlery in each hand — perhaps a spoon and fork or knife and fork? How does he hold cutlery — in his fist or between his thumb and fingers? Do you usually mash his food? Do you always cut up his food for him or can he cut some foods himself?
6. Please describe some of the foods he does not like.

(*Analysis of the list will give an indication of the types of food, if any, with which the child has difficulty. Dislike of slippery foods such as egg or jelly suggest that he has difficulty using his tongue to move food around in his mouth. Dislike of fibrous foods such as meat, some salad and vegetable items suggests that he has not developed an adequate chewing pattern.*)

7. Are there any difficulties when your child drinks? Does he drink from a bottle? Does he put his hands on it?

(*A child who can do so is able to put his hands together in mid-line.*)

Does he drink from a cup with a spout? Is he able to drink from a conventional cup? Is he able to hold it himself and lift it to his lips? Is he able to grade how much liquid reaches his mouth or does he often tip over the cup? Is he able to put the cup down without spilling the contents?

Washing

1. Where do you bath your child? In the bath? In a baby bath? In

the kitchen sink or washbasin? Does he lie or sit?
2. Do you need to support him while he is being bathed?
3. Does he have a special seat or support in the bath?
4. Do you think that he feels safe in the bath? Does he prefer to hold the bath sides or grab rails?
5. Does he co-operate when you bath him, for instance giving you an arm or leg to wash? Is he able to wash some parts of himself? Is he able to wash himself independently?
6. Do you have any difficulties brushing his teeth? Does he gag when you brush his back teeth? Does he tend to bite the toothbrush? (*Very often children who suffer from cerebral palsy have these types of difficulty*.)
Is he able to make some attempt at brushing his own teeth? Does he have difficulty making the necessary small repeated brushing movements? Can you rely on him to brush his teeth effectively?

Toilet

1. Is your child dry during the day? Is he dry at night? Is he clean?
2. Does he indicate when he wants to use the toilet? Do you have to judge when he needs to?
3. Does he sit on a potty? Does the potty need to be in a special place, for instance, in the corner of the room so that the walls give him some support? Does he have a special potty or a potty chair?
4. Is he able to sit on the toilet? Does he have a child size toilet seat insert? Do you need to hold him while he is sitting on the toilet?
5. Can he go to the toilet independently? Can he pull his pants down? Can he wipe himself?

Dressing

1. In what position do you dress and undress your child? On your lap? On the floor or on a bed? Does your child sit or stand?
2. Are any garments difficult to manage, for example, nappies or the sleeves of garments?
(*Spasticity often causes such difficulties, for example adductor spasm of the hip joint and flexor spasm of the elbow*.)
3. Does he co-operate when you are dressing him? Does he offer a foot when he sees you holding a sock or shoe, or an arm when he sees you holding a sleeve?

(*The questions about independence begin with undressing because children usually learn to take off before they are able to put on.*)
4. Can your child take off or begin to take off any of his clothes? Does it depend on what type of clothing he is wearing?
5. In what position is he when he undresses? Lying on the floor? Sitting on a stool or chair? Standing up?
(*The answers to these questions will indicate the child's balancing skills. A child who can undress while sitting is able to balance in that position without holding the chair with his hands. A child who is able to remove foot wear in a standing position is able to balance on one leg.*)
6. Can he put any garments on? Can he put garments on which go over his head?
(*Children who have spatial difficulties frequently have problems putting on garments which go over the head because they are unable to visually monitor their movements and the relationship of themselves to garments.*)
Can he put garments on the lower half of his body?
7. Can he manage buttons? Buckles? Zips? Shoe laces?
(*Difficulties with fastenings may be due to poor fine motor ability, lack of power, perceptual difficulties or mental impairment. Remediation will therefore depend on the cause of the problem.*)
8. Does your child sometimes refuse to get dressed even though you know he is able to manage the garments he is to wear?
(*Children for whom dressing requires more than the average amount of effort are often reluctant to try. Parents of these children should be advised to choose garments for their children which are easy to put on, of ample size, made of stretchy fabrics and with a minimum of fastenings. It is often better not to begin a 'battle' on occasions where there is a limited amount of time for dressing, for example, mornings when the child must arrive punctually at school. There are times, of course, when any child, including those with disabilities, will be reluctant to dress even though this is usually done without complaint. It can be difficult to decide if the child with disability is having real physical or emotional problems with dressing or is simply behaving awkwardly as do all children at times.*

Play

1. Does your child look at toys which you present to him? Does he follow them with his eyes if you move them? Is he attracted to toys

which make a noise?
2. Does he reach for toys with his hand? Does he reach more with one hand than the other?
(*Reaching more often with the left or right hand may indicate early hand preferences or the use of one hand to the exclusion of the other may indicate a deficit in the other as in hemiparesis.*)
3. In what position does he like to play? Lying on his tummy or back? Sitting on the floor or in a chair? Squatting or kneeling? Standing?
4. How does he play with toys? Hold them and look at them? Watch them as he manipulates them with two hands? Put them in his mouth? Hold a toy in either hand and bang them together? Transfer them from one hand to the other? Throw them? Pat them? Rake them?
5. Does he search for a toy which has fallen out of sight or which you have covered up?
(*Does the child appreciate the constancy of objects?*)
6. What are his favourite toys? Does he enjoy construction toys? Does he prefer to watch mechanical or electronic toys? Does he enjoy pretend play, playing at 'houses' or 'shops'? Does he like to help with domestic jobs or copy what you are doing? Does he enjoy playing outside, running about, digging in the garden or sand and on swings and slides?
(*Children who are nervous of playground equipment frequently have body image and spatial problems.*)
7. Does he enjoy playing alone? Do you often need to suggest play activities? Does he like you to play with him for most of the time?
8. Does he enjoy being with other children? Does he join in play activities with them or does he just play along-side them?

Independence skills

(*These questions only apply to children of such age and maturity where increasing independence is desirable.*)
1. Is your child able to make a cold drink for himself? A hot drink?
2. Is he able to make a snack for himself, perhaps a sandwich or beans on toast? Does he help you when you are preparing a meal?
(*The degree of independence a child has in the kitchen depends not only on his physical and mental abilities but also on how much he has learned by helping in the kitchen. Families differ in their attitudes to children helping, some feel that it is too dangerous whilst*

others encourage participation.)

3. Does your child understand money? Could he visit a nearby shop and make a purchase? Could he check if he had been given the correct change? Could he remember two or three items or would you need to write a note for the shopkeeper?
4. Does your child know how to cross a road? Could you rely on him to cross a small road safely?
5. Does he take part in any activities outside school such as Cubs, Scouts or other such associations?
6. Is he able to answer the telephone? Can he make a phone call from home? From a public call box?
7. Is he able to use public transport independently?

Parents will also engage in discussion about their child with the occupational therapist. As with any mode of questioning care should be taken not to pose loaded questions which give any indication of the best answer. Do not, for instance, ask 'does your child use a knife and fork to eat his dinner?' It suggests that the questioner expects an affirmative answer. The invitation 'Tell me how your child eats his dinner', does not presume any expected behaviour and leaves the parents free to describe their child's eating habits. As far as possible the child's abilities should be elicited in the latter manner so that parents feel free to present an honest picture of their child's behaviour at home.

Every therapist who is also a parent will know that it is not possible to paint a completely objective picture of one's own child; it is impossible where there is such close emotional involvement. Parents may underestimate their child's abilities and insist on helping when it is no longer necessary; others may overestimate abilities and feel disappointment when their child does not reach their expectations. Sometimes there is over-optimism about a child's abilities and potential which is obvious to everyone except the parents. The converse may also occur where parents adopt a destructively negative attitude which is unconsciously conveyed to the child. The experienced therapist will discern these and other attitudes and separate them from the facts of the child's behaviour.

The child too, if he is able to express himself, will provide valuable information about his abilities and difficulties and his attitudes towards them. The child who describes his hobbies as watching television and listening to his cassette or record player may well have motor difficulties which preclude precise gross or fine motor activities. The child who says that he does not like meat, fibrous vegetables and apples and pears unless they are peeled, should be suspected of having chewing difficulties. The child who likes playing with Lego, inset boards and other toys which provide limits of right and wrong but does not enjoy drawing may have problems with motor organisation. Listen to his likes and dislikes as they often provide indications of areas of ability which should be investigated.

Children, too, may be unrealistic regarding their abilities, both under- and over-estimating them. These attitudes may depend on their personalities or they may be used as devices to enable them to cope with their difficulties. Some children will describe their athletic prowess when investigation of their motor and perceptual skills suggests that they will have problems with physical activities. Other children who have very minor difficulties may describe their dissatisfaction with their own performance in various areas of the school curriculum.

The subjective comments of children and their parents are important parts of any assessment particularly when they are combined with the objective evidence elicited by the occupational therapist.

OBJECTIVE INFORMATION

From the moment of meeting the occupational therapist will be gathering information about the child and his family. She will notice his posture, gait, facial expression, his level of alertness, his awareness of his environment, his curiosity regarding the contents of the room.

Parents and their children have their own unique relationships and facets of it will be observable while they are with the occupational therapist.

1. Does the child cling to his mother or father, being reluctant even to sit at a table even a few feet away from them?
2. Does he fail to relate to them at all?
3. Is he over friendly with the therapist who is a stranger?
4. Does he respond to his parents' speech or do his parents use language well below his chronological age level when they address him, or do they use an unusually large number of gestures to reinforce speech? The last two strategies could indicate that parents are unconsciously adjusting to their child's poor comprehension of the spoken word.
5. When it is suggested that the child removes his coat or sweater

do his parents rush to help him when he is of an age when he should be able to do the task independently? Does the child wait for his parents to remove his clothing? This is perhaps the best indication of what usually happens at home.

The tasks which are set for the child will depend upon his apparent developmental age level (if this was immediately obvious there would be little need to set the tasks), his obvious impairments and his reported abilities. Whatever tasks are presented to him it will be possible to observe:

1. How he concentrates on the task
2. His interest in them.
3. His motivation and determination to succeed.
4. The sighted child will demonstrate his level of eye, concentration and, where manipulation skills are sufficiently developed, hand-eye co-ordination.
5. His problem-solving strategies.
6. With any level of task it will be possible to observe if the child is pleased and motivated by success or if he realises when he has failed and is upset by it.
7. Is the child content to repeat the same task over and over again if allowed to do so?
8. Is he eager to try the next task or is he apprehensive of unfamiliar ones?
9. Does he show the appropriate amount of displeasure if a toy with which he is playing is removed, or does he manipulate any toy which is put in his hands with equal enthusiasm or lack of interest?

The specific activities presented by the occupational therapist will depend on a number of criteria:

1. Her role in a particular clinical situation.
2. The physical and mental developmental level of the child.
3. The nature of his impairment.

Previous discussion will have elicited the child's particular likes and dislikes. Try to begin the formal part of the procedure with something the child enjoys doing. A drawing activity is often suitable particularly if it begins with the child's choice of subject. Other activities will be more suitable in specific situations but they should be those at which the child cannot 'fail', those in which there is no right or wrong.

Be sure to begin at a level well within the child's capabilities. It is better for the child to comment on the simplicity of the task and the occupational therapist to be in honest agreement than for the child to be deterred and discouraged from further co-operation because the task is beyond his developmental level or physical capabilities.

The occupational therapist will be involved in a number of areas of development and ability. She will almost always investigate hand function and perception. Both of these ranges of skills will be viewed in the light of the child's chronological age and his developmental level and his lifestyle. There are skills which are necessary in the life of most children in which hand function and perception are important parts. The occupational therapist should look at all these aspects of living:

1. Personal independence in keeping with his developmental level.
2. The ability to enjoy toys and other materials which are used for imaginative, symbolic, imitative and constructional play.
3. The ability to make the best use of formal educational facilities which are provided for him.

Exactly how the occupational therapist undertakes these observations will depend on the type of situation in which she is employed, her job description and the range of problems she encounters. The therapist who works, for instance, only with children suffering from JCA will probably choose more formal and precise initial procedures using detailed printed forms, whereas the therapist who works in a clinic that sees all children of all ages suffering from continuity impairments will probably find it impossible to formulate a form which will suit every child.

Observations of the use of bricks

Bricks are, perhaps, the most versatile pieces of assessment equipment, which may be used with young babies and children up to a developmental age of about seven years to assess motor and perceptual skills. Standard 2.5 cm wooden bricks of various colours should be used. A minimum of twelve will be required, two of each of six colours. Most of the activities useful for assessment may be successfully demonstrated without the need for verbal instructions so they may be used with children who have difficulty comprehending the spoken word or who suffer from severe deafness.

Beginning with the assessment of young babies the bricks may be used in the following ways.

1. Notice the baby's interest in bricks which are set out before him. Observe if he scans the entire array.
2. Note any movement he makes to reach for the bricks. At a

developmental level of 16 weeks the baby will attempt to reach for a brick. At a 20 week level he will be able to grasp one with a palmar grip.

3. Notice his behaviour when a second brick is offered. At a 24 week level he will drop the first brick when a second one is offered. Four weeks later he will be able to hold one brick in each hand with a thumb and fingers grip.

4. At a 40 week level he will adopt an index finger approach when reaching for a brick. He will not yet be able to release the brick voluntarily. He may try to press the heel of his hand on a hard surface to facilitate release.

5. Interest usually develops first in taking objects out of a container, a little later he will begin putting things into one. Success will depend on the stability of the container, its dimensions and the size of the aperture.

6. Casting usually begins at the developmental age of one year (and has usually stopped by about an 18 month level). In order to do this the child must be able to release them though he will not be able to grade the movement: it will be an all or nothing movement. He will hold a brick between his index finger and thumb.

7. During the first year the manipulation of bricks will indicate the child's level of motor development as well as any deviant behaviour. It will be possible to observe if he 'ignores' one hand and refuses to reach and grasp with it. Spasticity in the form of a splayed approach to the bricks may be noticed as may any unsteadiness or tremor which may result from athetosis or ataxia.

8. At a 15 month level the child will be able to put one brick on top of another. The number of bricks he can build will increase until at three years he will be able to build a tower nine bricks high. It is not sufficient to record how many bricks high a child is able to build; notes should be made regarding how he does it. To be successful he must be able to co-ordinate hand and eye and to concentrate on the task. A child who persists in his use of a palmar grasp will be unable to place bricks on top of each other accurately, as will the child who cannot grade release. Involuntary movements will prevent placement and may also disturb those bricks which have already been built.

9. Children who have the manipulative skills necessary may be asked to build other structures. A 'train' consisting of a row of three bricks plus a fourth brick on top of the first will be constructed by most children who have reached a two and a half year level. At a three year level the child will imitate a 'bridge' built with two bricks

Figure 8.1: A four brick train, a three brick bridge and six brick steps

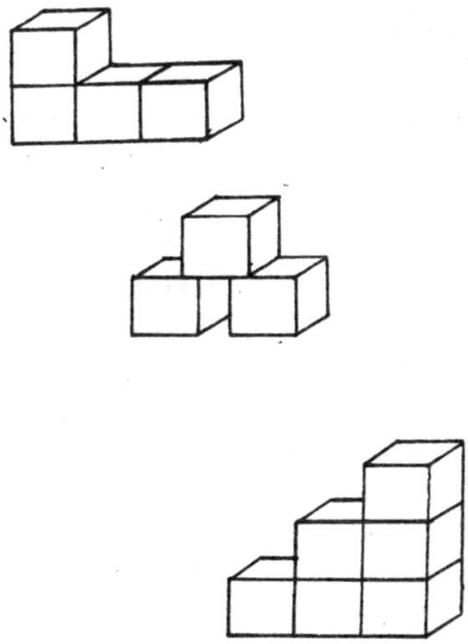

with a space between them and a third brick placed on top. At about a five year level the child will copy 'steps' constructed with rows of three, two and one brick (see Figure 8.1). By observing the child's attempts to build these structures it will be possible to observe his perceptual skills of the spatial relationships of objects.

10. Bricks may also be used to observe the child's sense of colour which develops through three stages.

(a) Matching colours.
(b) Selecting those which have been named.
(c) Naming colours.

Begin at the lowest level of matching colours, showing the child a brick and asking him to select a similar coloured one from the array in front of him. Should he not understand the verbal request, demonstrate what you would like him to do. Progress through all the colours available in case he is only able to match one or two of the colours. If the child is able to match colours progress to selecting named ones by asking the child to give you a brick of a particular named colour, 'Give me a red one', etc. Again, try all the colours as the child may only understand verbal labels for a few of the colours which are presented. If this stage is successful progress to asking the child to name the colours of the bricks. Children begin to be able to name colours at about three and a half year level and can usually name primary and intermediate shades by the time they have reached a five year level. Red and yellow are often the first colours the child is able to name while confusion with the blue and green frequently continues for some time.

11. Bricks may also be used to observe the child's concept of number: does he understand 'one and more than one'; does he understand two, three and four? Hold out your hand and ask the child to give you one brick. Do not give any sign of recognition when he has done so; leave your hand in place and wait to see if he offers you more. Many children are adept at reading the signs on the face of an adult when the correct number has been given when, in fact, they have little idea of number. Continue in this manner asking for larger numbers of bricks.

12. Putting the bricks away in their box together with the child is an additional useful activity for observing his hand skills. Note if he is able to hold more than one brick in his hand and whether he spontaneously employs both hands. Note if he is able to place the bricks in accurate rows or piles them up in a haphazard manner. Placing the last brick in a row requires a delicate finger thumb grip. Lastly is the child able to replace the lid of the box, a two-handed activity which requires it to be lowered in a symmetrical manner.

Observations of the use of formboards and posting boxes

These types of assessment equipment vary greatly in their degree of complexity, from having only one shape to be fitted into a single inset or hole to having a large number of shapes, symmetrical and asymmetrical, varying in size and shape. Begin assessment of ability with equipment which will be well within the child's ability so that initial success is certain.

These types of equipment measure:

1. Perceptual skills.
2. The matching of shapes to various insets or holes.
3. The relative size of pieces.
4. Their position in space and their relationships to each other.
5. For the child with manipulative difficulties there is the additional element of grasping.
6. Manoeuvring the pieces into the correct position in relation to the inset or hole.
7. Placing and releasing them.

The use of this equipment will therefore include the assessment

Figure 8.2: A selection of handles on pieces from a formboard requiring a two finger and thumb grip, a whole hand cylindrical grip and a pronated whole hand grip

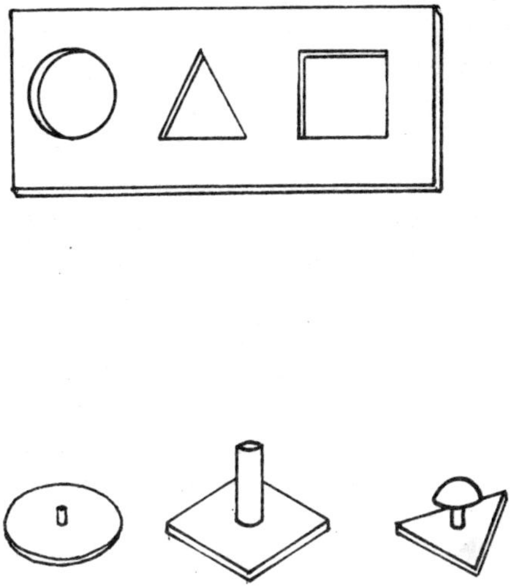

of both perceptual and motor skills. For some children it will not be appropriate to set time limits for their attempts to complete these tasks because of their impaired motor skills.

1. If necessary use formboards which have handles attached to each piece which enables the child with impaired grip to manipulate them. In some instances use a small knob which enables the child to adopt a thumb and two, three or four finger grip. Other children will need a large knob which can be held with an intermediate four finger or even a crude palmar grasp (see Figure 8.2).

2. It may not be possible or indeed appropriate to affix handles to the stock of formboards used for assessment. An alternative solution is to press a drawing pin into the centre of each piece so that it will attract a magnet. The child is provided with the magnet attached to a handle which he may grasp with a whole hand vertical grip or a magnet attached to a strap which is fastened with Velcro around the child's knuckles so that he may extract or place pieces using a flexed horizontal hand (see Figure 8.3).

3. Some children who have difficulty with grip and placement will manage to place pieces in insets if the pieces are considerably deeper than the insets so that he may retain his grip on the whole piece until it is located within the inset. This device will also aid release because

Table 8.3: A handle with a magnet for removing and replacing formboard pieces. A strap which fits round the hand to which a magnet is attached. It has a Velcro fastening

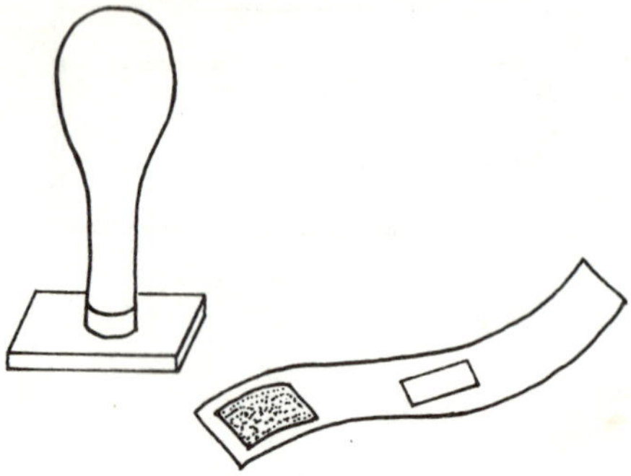

the lower part of the piece will be secured in the inset against a crude release.

4. Posting boxes test more or less the same skills as formboards though for the immobile child the former may create more difficulty because of their height and, in some models, their lack of stability.

5. Care should be taken in the choice of posting boxes to ensure that only those with unambiguous pieces are used. An example of such ambiguity is a box which contains pieces of spherical shape which passes through a round hole, a cylindrical shape which passes through a smaller round hole and a disc shape which must be passed through a rectangular slit. A child using such a box at home or playgroup would learn the placing of the various pieces, but it is not suitable for initial assessment.

6. An ideal type of box is one to which a graded variety of lids may be fitted so that the task may be varied from placing a single shape, placing two or three symmetrical shapes to placing four or more irregular unfamiliar shapes (see Figure 8.4). Thus the therapist will be able to assess the child's grip, placement and release, his ability to understand the concept of 'putting in', his ability to match simple shapes and align them with the appropriate holes and to appreciate the asymmetry of irregular shapes, match and align them with the appropriate insets. Such boxes also allow the therapist to begin at a level where the child will succeed.

(a) At about a 15 month level the average child will be able to place a round piece.

(b) After some trial and error a child will place a circle, square

Figure 8.4: Posting box with a number of lids so that the difficulty of the task may be finely graded

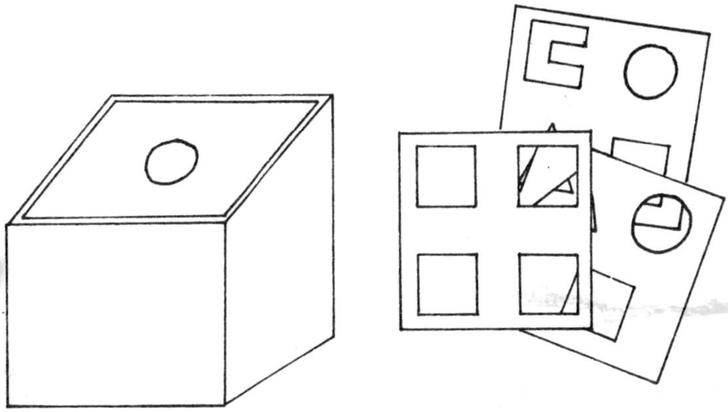

and triangle when he has reached a two year level.
(c) At a three year level he will place all three without trial and error.
(d) At a three and a half year level the average child will be able to complete a ten piece formboard containing a variety of geometric shapes in about one minute.
(e) Such an activity will also indicate to the therapist how well the child is able to concentrate on a task and how well he is able to scan the table for appropriate pieces.

Crayons and pencils

At a 15 month level a child will make a mark on paper *if he is given the opportunity to do so*. This is a very important point; the occupational therapist should always inquire, if the child is pre-school age and particularly if he does not attend a nursery or playgroup, whether he has been given crayons or pencils and paper at home. It does not occur to some parents that a very young child may enjoy scribbling and others are afraid that their child will damage furnishings or wallpaper.

Have ready a variety of drawing implements including crayons, pencils, felt-tip pens and chalks, because children vary in the type of drawing tool they can best manage according to their motor skills and previous experience at home. Do not assume that the younger the child the thicker the crayon or pencil he will prefer; some very young children manipulate a thin implement best. Some children prefer short stubby crayons, others a long slim pencil.

Drawing activities will provide the occupational therapist with information about:

1. Fine motor skills, including, of course, the development of his pencil grip.
2. Eye-hand co-ordination.
3. Praxis or ability to organise his movements.
4. Perceptual skills.

Drawing is often a good activity with which to begin an assessment; if the child is allowed his own choice of subject in the first instance he cannot make errors, he is sure of success and the session will begin in a relaxed manner. Unless the subject of the drawing is obvious it is wise not to interrogate the child too closely about it. Certainly do not ask the child what he has drawn; young children frequently do not attempt to draw anything in particular and will only define their efforts to please adults. I have observed a number of children who have motor difficulties who will draw and then suggest that there drawing looks like a particular object indicating that they made marks on the paper first and then decided what it could represent.

From this initial free choice drawing it will be possible to note some of the following points.

1. The hand in which the child prefers to hold his pencil. Some very young children will try one hand and then the other, though most will demonstrate a preference. Children who have a motor deficit on one side, hemiparesis or other forms of cerebral palsy where one hand is more affected than the other, or a slight impairment of one side which is often associated with clumsiness or incoordination, may draw with first one hand and then the other. This behaviour is often due to the child's innate preferred hand being the least able one. In this situation the child instinctively wishes to use his least able hand but at the same time knows that the function of the other is superior. It may be some time before a child consistently holds a pencil in the same hand. Given the time and opportunity to experiment he will usually make the best decision for himself.
2. The type of pencil grip he adopts. The stages in the development of pencil grip usually proceed as follows:

(a) The very young child holds the pencil or crayon with a whole hand supinated ulnar grip, using whole arm movements to mark the paper.
(b) Next the hand is held in pronation still adopting a whole hand grip.
(c) The index finger extends down the shaft of the pencil or crayon.
(d) At the developmental level of two and a half years the average child is developing a tripod grip involving the pads of the thumb and index finger and the radial side of the distal phalanx of the middle finger.
(e) This type of grip usually continues to develop until at a seven year level the grip is said to be 'dynamic' when intrinsic muscle activity is present.

3. Some children do not spontaneously adopt a dynamic tripod grip, sometimes because they copy the grip used by a parent but more often because of motor impairment. The child with spasticity often holds his pencil with a flexed finger grip; tremor or ataxia may counteract it by spreading the index, middle and ring fingers down the shaft of the pencil. The child with arthrogryposis, or other conditions, which prevent flexion of the fingers, may spontaneously hold his pencil in the cleft between two extended fingers.
4. The posture the child adopts in relation to the table and paper will provide an indication of difficulties which will affect not only writing and drawing but other fine motor activities. The persistent adoption of an asymmetrical posture, particularly if the child also fails to support his paper with the non-drawing hand frequently occurs in hemiparesis.
5. The quality of the marks the child makes on the paper will provide clues to some of the motor problems from which the child may suffer. A tremor, ataxia or athetosis may be observable in the child's movements but will also be evident in the pencil strokes he makes. The child whose hand movements lack power will make faint marks on the paper. A selection of a child's drawings over a period of time will provide a record of his progress with or deterioration of his hand control.

Drawing lines and geometric shapes

Provided that children have been given the opportunity to practise pencil skills, their ability usually follows a predictable pattern. In the early years children do differ in their interests and some children are not interested in drawing and colouring until they are approaching school age. Once their interest is stimulated they usually progress rapidly until their skills are commensurate with their peers who have already enjoyed using pencils and crayons for some time. Should the child who is being assessed be reluctant to draw other methods should be devised to estimate his fine hand skills.

The drawing skills of the average child develop in the following order.

1. At an 18 month level the child will imitate a crayon stroke.
2. At a two year level he will imitate a vertical stroke which has been demonstrated to him. His attempt is counted as successful if it is within 30 degrees of the vertical.
3. At a two and a half year level he will imitate a horizontal stroke which will be within 30 degrees of the horizontal. The child who has difficulty controlling his crayon will probably draw the initial stroke satisfactorily but he may have difficulty removing his crayon from the paper cleanly and as a result the end of the stroke will tail off downwards towards the child.
4. At a three year level the child will be able to imitate a cross. To do so he must be able to organise his movements efficiently in both a vertical and horizontal direction and in relation to the first line which has been drawn. He must also be able to perceive the relationship of the two lines to each other. He will also be able to imitate a circle which is demonstrated to him. To be successful his circle must demonstrate circularity and be joined reasonably accurately.
5. A square is the first shape which requires the child to make a change of direction while his crayon remains on the paper. The average child will be successful at copying a square when he has reached a four to four and a half year level. The child who is unable to make these 90 degree changes of direction will probably represent the shape with four separate lines arranged in a square shape. The method of construction of the square should be recorded in a precise manner so that his difficulties may be analysed in order to prepare appropriate treatment plans.
6. A triangle is the first geometric shape which children are asked to draw which contains diagonal lines. They are usually successful at about a five year level. The example with which the child is presented should be an equilateral triangle, not a right angled triangle, so that it contains two diagonal lines. Children who have difficulty with diagnosis will either round the top of the triangle to make the lines meet or draw a right angle and attempt to join these

two lines together. Children who have difficulty with this shape frequently experience particular difficulty with the formation of letter characters such as *y*, *w*, *s* and *k*.

7. Children reach a developmental level of between six and seven years before they are able to draw a diamond. They can usually draw the top half of it before they are able to complete the bottom half. To be acceptable the shape should not be simply a square rotated through 45 degrees, it must have top and bottom angles of less than 90 degrees and the two angles at the sides more than 90 degrees.

Drawing a human figure

Children who have reached a developmental level of three years will draw a simple representation of a human figure. Some will attempt to do so before they reach this level, others will be reluctant to attempt to draw a person if they are not confident that they will succeed.

If the child has been allowed to produce drawings of his own choice at the beginning of the assessment session, the occupational therapist may be able to use these drawings to lead the child towards the drawings she needs for evaluation purposes. For example, if the child has drawn a car or a lorry the occupational therapist could encourage the child to draw the driver or she could ask the child to draw the people who live in the house, play in the garden or on the beach which the child has drawn.

In order to draw a human figure the child must possess the skills already described and he must also understand the relationships of the parts of the human figure. If the child has been successful with other drawing tasks but fails to produce a human figure in keeping with the other skills he has demonstrated, further observations should be made regarding the child's understanding of his own and other people's bodies.

The resultant drawing may be scored on the Goodenough 'Draw-a-Man' Test which awards points for the various details included in the drawing, such as head and legs being present and the width of the eyes being greater than their height. The precise method of scoring is listed in *The Development of the Infant and Young Child: Normal and Abnormal*, by R.S. Illingworth and in the *Aston Index*, by Margaret Newton and Michael Thomson (Newton and Thomson, 1976). The test is primarily a measure of intelligence and is said to correlate well with the Binet tests (Illingworth, 1980, p. 234).

Personal experience indicates that children who have minor motor problems will not be penalised in this test by their poor drawing ability — it is not measuring artistic ability — but on the details of the human figure which are drawn. Sometimes a child will indicate his own physical disability in his drawing, hemiplegia being indicated by one side of the body being smaller and less defined than the other or spina bifida by the lower half of the drawing being disproportionately small although this is not always the case.

Care should be taken when using the contents of the drawings of older children, particularly those over ten years, for assessment purposes because children tend to take on adult attitudes towards drawing the human figure and become inhibited and reluctant to express themselves. As the child matures drawing also becomes stylised so that detail of which the child is well aware is omitted and scoring the drawing produces an underestimate of his level of ability.

9

Assessment and Treatment Plans

Understanding human needs is half the job of meeting them.
Adlai Stevenson (1952)

From the subjective and objective observations the occupational therapist will form opinions, make estimates, evaluate the child's strengths and weaknesses. She will weigh the observations of the child and his parents with how she has observed the child performing and draw up a plan of how the child can best be helped. She will evolve probable reasons for the child's difficulties on which to base her treatment plan.

The subjective observations of the child and his parents are likely to be of a practical nature. A child may say that he does not enjoy drawing and colouring, he prefers playing with his cars and garage. His parents may comment that though he has been in school eight months he does not seem interested in writing his name and his attempts are hardly recognisable as such. The occupational therapist may have observed him building a tower of 2.5 cm bricks and recorded that his tower was only five high; she knows that most children can build to this height by the time they are two years old and that the average child of three would build nine bricks high. She will have noted the level of concentration on the task, his interest in it, his hand-eye co-ordination. She may have noticed that as the tower of cubes became higher and his forearm was no longer supported by the table that a slight tremor was apparent. On examining his drawing she may discern slight unsteadiness in the lines he has drawn. This unsteadiness may also have been apparent when he was placing small pegs in a pegboard. There may also have been imprecision in his finger-thumb grip making the insertion of the pegs in the board difficult.

It is likely that the child will also have an unorthodox pencil grip, he may spread his fingers up the shaft of the pencil in an attempt to gain more stability or he may have the index and middle finger on top of the pencil with hyperextension of the distal interphalangeal joint and his thumb tending to drift across it. It is becoming clear why this child prefers to play with cars and garage which require only gross hand function and with which there is no right or wrong.

Are there additional reasons for his difficulty with writing his name; perhaps he can trace over the letters quite effectively but is unable to form them free hand. Are his parents recorded as saying he has difficulty fastening buttons in spite of repeated instruction? It seems likely that he also has difficulty with motor organisation planning movements required for daily living activities.

Thus the picture of his skills and difficulties may be pieced together using both subjective and objective evidence. In this way not only does the therapist gain insight into the nature of the child's problems but also his parents learn why there is difficulty with certain tasks, that their child is not being awkward or stubborn but that there are reasons for his problems. Together plans can be made to remedy the difficulties or to find ways around them.

Above is just one example of some of the difficulties of one child. His assessment would of course encompass every area of difficulty and how his problems impinged on his development and every aspect of life.

Many children who are referred to an occupational therapist will suffer from much more severe and intractable impairments: some will suffer from degenerative conditions and others will never be able to live an independent life. There will be a few sad instances where little can be done for the child but where treatment will be directed towards helping the parents care for the child more easily.

Case note

Georgina is a severely handicapped child who suffers from microcephalus, resultant severe mental handicap and cerebral palsy. She makes no response to people or her environment, her only response is a reflex one to being tickled. Her mother is remarkable in the way she lovingly cares for her physical needs and the gentle way in which she continues to talk to her even though Georgina makes no response.

The main problems with care are her sleeping position, her tightly flexed hands and her inability to sit securely in her pushchair. It is best for her to sleep on her side but after being placed in this position she falls over on to her back and wakens. The problem was solved by providing a foam gutter in which she is held in a side-lying position.

In order to maintain a good position in her pushchair a lightweight thermoplastic inset was modelled with head pieces which maintain her head in mid line.

Because she held her hands tightly flexed they were difficult to wash and the palmar skin was affected by an accumulation of perspiration. Thermoplastic hand splints were made but in spite of firm straps her hands gradually reverted to a tightly flexed position. Extension was achieved when the splints were modified by cutting a slit at the metacarpophalangeal joint through which her fingers were passed. The splint then covered the dorsum of the forearm and the palmar aspect of the hand and fingers.

Nothing positive has been achieved to aid Georgina's development but these devices have simplified handling for her mother.

Where the occupational therapy assessment is one of a number which will be undertaken it is important that the several individual assessments are considered together so that the child and his parents are provided with one overall plan for their child. Families can so easily be overburdened with seemingly conflicting advice and individual plans from each therapist involved with their child.

Sometimes children are referred for one specific treatment need. An example of this would be the child suffering from JCA who is referred for the provision of orthoses. Such a referral entails more than the making of splints; it also includes discovering how the child feels about needing to wear them and how his parents feel because their attitudes can influence their effective use. Discussion regarding orthoses often leads to discussion of how the child and his family feel about the prolonged disease. The point being that whatever the condition the occupational therapist must consider the whole child, his development and his lifestyle and that of his family when making her assessment.

Case note

Carol, who suffers from JCA, was referred at two and a half years for the provision of night-resting splints. Her very young parents were understandably extremely concerned about their daughter's condition. This anxiety was transferred to Carol which together with her general feeling of malaise made her a very apprehensive client.

The splints were prepared ready for fitting and, because she was so young, her therapist enquired if Carol liked to go to sleep sucking her thumb. Carol did suck her thumb. Holding up the splint complete with thumb piece the occupational therapist said, 'I'll cut it off then'. Not realising that the therapist was referring to the splint and not her thumb, Carol ran screaming to her mother. How important, particularly with young apprehensive children, that words are chosen carefully!

After being reassured, she had her splint fitted. Because of recurring flare-ups of her condition it was particularly important that she practised her exercise regime regularly at home and that it was supervised by her physiotherapist. Unfortunately she associated physiotherapy with pain and discomfort and could not be persuaded to co-operate with her. It was an example of the occupational therapist needing to take over the role of another therapist for the benefit of the client.

As the disease progressed Carol also required working hand splints and, at times, night leg splints to encourage full extension of the knees. She was co-operative when having them measured, fitted and adjusted. The soiled condition of them when she returned for check-ups supported her parents reports that she was happy to wear them.

One further problem remained — when Carol was comparatively well, she failed to attend appointments. Her parents needed much counselling before they understood the need to continue treatment even though their daughter seemed well. When they realised the importance of maintaining the full range of joint movement and building muscle power to protect joints they became regular in their attendance despite her father working shifts and a family bereavement.

Whatever the child's condition and his parents' attitudes it is important that they leave after the assessment with something positive however small. The child should have acquired at least a small element of a new skill or have demonstrated a new interest, or his parents given some practical advice about handling or loaned a necessary piece of equipment. The assessment must be concluded with an item of positive help.

It is easy to consider the job completed once the child has been assessed. This is rarely the case: in the field of paediatrics the therapist is dealing with a situation in which there are many variables. The condition of childhood implies that further physical and mental development has yet to occur. There will be changes in the child's size and weight, in neurology, in his perceptual and intellectual skills and in his emotional behaviour. Family situations change as do parental attitudes. Previous assessment records must be constantly reviewed so that treatment plans are geared to current problems.

TREATMENT PLANS

How, where, when and by whom a child will receive treatment will depend upon his medical and social history, the subjective and objective data which has been gathered and the assessment which has been made of that data. Plans must be made for each individual child, for though the physical or mental problems of two or more children may be almost identical, their life situations almost certainly will not be.

Case note

At the age of ten months, Jack was diagnosed to be suffering from Erb's Palsy; the diagnosis was subsequently revised to one of left hemiparesis. A brain scan revealed a mild degree of arrested hydrocephalus. At three years he was seen by an educational psychologist who estimated his IQ to be in the low average range. His orthoptist diagnosed hemianopia.

Combined physiotherapy and occupational therapy sessions were planned.

The aims of his treatment were:

1. To make Jack aware of his left side.
2. Because of his hemianopia to encourage him to turn his head to look at his left hand.
3. To encourage bilateral activities.
4. To encourage extension of both arms.
5. To encourage the use of the left hand and arm as stabilisers.
6. To encourage extension of his left hand.

The behavioural objectives of his treatment were planned as follows.

1. He will have bells and other noisy toys attached to his left wrist.
2. He will sit at a table with a cut out so that both his hands are in view on the table. Toys will be presented from the left so that he turns to look at that side and thus his left hand.
3. He will play with large toys such as beach balls which necessitate the use of both hands and arms to hold them. He will be presented with heavy toys which necessitate the use of both hands to carry

them. He will play with unstable toys such as Kelly dolls which require the use of his left hand to stabilise them.
4. He will play reciprocal games with his occupational therapist and members of his family using a heavy medicine ball or a large cylinder necessitating the extension of both arms for pushing them away from himself.
5. He will make prints of his left hand on a large sheet of paper on a table. He will stand so that printing involves not only extension of the hand but also of the wrist and elbow.

When treatment began Jack's parents had just separated following five years of stormy, sometimes physically violent, marriage. His mother was coping alone with Jack and his older sister, living in a council house in a very rough area of the city. She resented living in the area in which she had been allocated a house and found it difficult to manage financially on her social security benefit. At one point she became extremely depressed and attempted suicide.

Her attendance with her son for treatment was erratic. When they did attend she was nervous and, despite the therapists' attempts to build rapport, her attitude remained very much one of 'us and them'. She adopted a pleading attitude towards her son and her tone suggested that she did not really expect him to co-operate. The therapists felt that she was stretched to her limits coping with her personal problems, her home and her children. There was little carry over to the home of treatment suggestions demonstrated to her at the clinic.

The first five years of Jack's education were at the local primary school, after which he transferred to a school for children with physical handicaps. This move was necessary because of Jack's attitude towards his physical disability rather than its severity.

He returned for occupational therapy assessment at the age of 14 years. He was almost completely dependent on his mother for self-care and the activities of daily living. He has no personal friends, lacks self-esteem and social life outside the home.

Case note

James' hemiparesis was not formally diagnosed until he was three years old, although it had been present since birth. His parents had been instinctively treating it since it became apparent that he was reluctant to use his right hand when he was a few months old. They had drawn his attention to that hand and encouraged a bilateral approach to large toys.

His consultant referred him for full team assessment: he was found to have an IQ in the average range and there was no visual involvement. The physiotherapist found him to have a tight tendo Achilles of the right leg which she treated with serial plasters and exercise; later he was fitted with a thermo-plastic ankle foot orthosis.

The occupational therapist found that he tackled activities with a left-handed approach wherever possible and that the right hand was held in flexion with the thumb adducted across the palm. With effort he was able to extend his wrist and fingers and attain some abduction of his thumb. His drawing skills were found to be below his chronological age level.

The aims of his treatment were:

1. To encourage extension of the wrist and fingers of the right hand.
2. To encourage abduction of the right thumb.
3. To encourage the use of the right hand as a helping and stabilising hand.
4. To encourage the development of his drawing skills.

The behavioural objectives of his treatment were planned as follows.

1. (a) When drawing, James will support the paper with his extended right hand.
   (b) When drawing on a floor chalk board, he will kneel up, support himself with his extended right hand and arm, thus bearing weight through it from shoulder to hand.
   (c) Using thick powder paint he will make prints of his hands.
   (d) When his mother has been making pastry he will be given the scraps to roll out using an adult-sized rolling pin.
   (e) When playing ball together with his father, a large ball will be used so that James uses both hands to catch it.
   (f) He will play 'wheel barrows' with his parents thus bearing weight through his arms and hands.
2. He will wear a leather figure-of-eight splint to hold his thumb in abduction.
3. (a) He will steady stacking barrels with his right hand while he opens them with his left hand.
   (b) He will steady a musical box with his right hand while he winds it up with his left hand.
   (c) He will steady a Jack-in-the-box with his right hand while he presses the button to release Jack with his left hand.
4. (a) He will place pegs in a pegboard thus encouraging the development of a precise finger thumb grip.

(b) He will play with a lacing toy holding the end of the lace in his left hand with a precise finger thumb grip.
(c) He will draw using a pencil fitted with a triangular grip, having his thumb on one face of it, index finger on the next face and middle finger under the pencil on the third face of the triangular grip.
(d) He will draw inside stencils of shapes appropriate to his developmental level so that he knows the 'feel' of the movement when he draws them.

Though James lived 20 miles from the clinic he attended regularly for his fortnightly appointments. His parents conscientiously encouraged regular practice of his occupational therapy techniques at home. When he reached school age his occupational therapist explained the nature of his difficulties and his treatment programme to his teacher who was constructively sympathetic to his difficulties. She encouraged him to try the same activities as the other children in her class but appreciated his limitations. Because of his early difficulties with pencil control he received extra attention during handwriting lessons.

James is now ten years old and visits his occupational therapist three times a year when his progress is reviewed. He is now coping well with handwriting, is popular with his peers and well adjusted to his residual disability.

Plans of treatment must clearly be geared towards the needs and capabilities of each child and his family. Realistic plans must be made taking into account the child's personality, the attitudes of his family and the nature of his impairments.

Where the treatment takes place will depend on a number of factors: the purpose of the treatment; the mobility of the child's family, the mobility of the occupational therapist and the amount of time available to her.

Treatment in a clinic

Advantages

1. The full range of occupational therapy equipment is immediately available.
2. It is an economical use of the occupational therapist's time because she does not spend time travelling.
3. It is a good place to carry out standardised tests because the

environment can be controlled.

Disadvantages

1. Children and parents may spend a considerable amount of time travelling to a clinic, particularly if they use public transport. This point is particularly important if treatments are to continue over a prolonged period.
2. The occupational therapist does not see the child in a real life situation, which is particularly important when dressing or feeding difficulties are being treated.
3. A clinic, especially if it is situated within a hospital, suggests sickness even though most of the children treated by the occupational therapist will not be acutely or chronically sick.
4. Older children may resent frequent absences from school to visit a clinic. They may be embarrassed by peers questioning them regarding the reasons for their frequent absences from school.

Treatment at home

Advantages

1. The child and his family will be more relaxed meeting the occupational therapist on their own territory.
2. The occupational therapist will be able to observe the domestic circumstances of the family and plan her treatment accordingly.
3. Home visits save the family time and money.

Disadvantages

1. Home visits are expensive in therapist time.
2. Some families are not happy for professionals to visit their homes.
3. Some children may find it difficult to concentrate on therapy in a house where siblings are playing.

Treatment in school or nursery

Advantages

1. The occupational therapist is able to observe children and discuss with staff problems which are peculiar to school or nursery.
2. Meeting with teachers and nursery staff allows the occupational therapist to explain the aims of treatment and exchange observations on the child.

Disadvantages

1. Such visits are expensive in therapist time.
2. Some children may be embarrassed or resent being singled out as different by their occupational therapist seeing them in nursery or school.
3. There may not be a room or quiet area available in which to carry out treatment.

The frequency and length of treatment sessions

Very few occupational therapists work in perfect situations where they have unlimited time in which to treat children, where parents have no difficulty attending for appointments and teachers and nursery staff can easily accommodate the needs of the occupational therapist. The frequency and length of therapy sessions must take into account a number of variables.

The occupational therapist

The frequency of treatment sessions will be limited to some extent by the occupational therapist's work load and the number of hours which she has available for treatment. Those who see children mainly in a clinical situation will have more time available for patient contact than those who travel to make school and home visits.

The family

The frequency of treatment will be affected by the ease with which the family travels to the clinic. The occupational therapist must always bear in mind that most of the children she sees will have continuing impairment which may require many years of therapy. Frequent visits for therapy in acute conditions are usually easily accommodated by most families; where treatment continues over a prolonged period the following possibilities should be considered:

1. Stress in the parent who usually attends with the child for therapy.
2. Tension between spouses because of the frequent absence of the one who escorts the child to therapy.
3. Ill-feeling between spouses because household duties are neglected.
4. Ill-feeling between spouses because extra attention is being given to the child with impairment.
5. Siblings jealous of the special attention given to the child with impairment.

6. Parents who are able to carry over the aims and objectives of occupational therapy into the daily life of the child will require fewer sessions with the occupational therapist than those who are unable to effect this carry over.

The child

1. The length of time for which the child is able to concentrate will sometimes dictate the length of treatment sessions. The child who can only concentrate for perhaps 20 minutes, would benefit from frequent short sessions. Conversely, other children may require a settling down period before they are able to concentrate on therapy. These points are particularly relevant to occupational therapy where the active co-operation of the child is necessary before purposeful activity may take place.
2. In some conditions it may be appropriate to plan treatment sessions in a series followed by a break. Such series of treatment are particularly suitable for school age children who can have intensive therapy during school holidays thus avoiding absences from school.
3. In some conditions, such as JCA, there will be periods when the disease is active and when intensive periods of therapy will be necessary.

Aims and objectives of treatment

An assessment which looks at every aspect of a child's life will allow the occupational therapist to draw up a list of problems which affect the child. Some problems will be solved immediately or in the near future and others may continue for months or years. The problems should be recorded for future reference and, so that they may be discussed, broken down into their components and solutions sought.

The solving of the elements of problems should then be set out as aims. For example, the child who has problems with handwriting will have the nature of his difficulties analysed (Alston and Taylor, 1984). Should one of his problems be forming letters in the correct manner, the general aim would be for him to form letters correctly. This aim would be broken down into short-term aims, one of which may be to learn how to form *c* shapes so that he may write the letters which begin with this shape.

General and specific behavioural objectives are also specified for the child. These describe what the child will *actually do*. Continuing the example of he child with handwriting problems the general

behavioural objective would be for the child to form letters correctly. Specific behavioural objectives would include:
1. The child will draw *c* shapes using a stencil.
2. The child will copy the movements of the therapist and he will draw a *c* shape.
3. The child will draw *c* shapes independently.
4. The child will draw *o*, *d*, *g*, *q*, *a* which all begin with a *c*.

Behavioural objectives always specify what the child will *actually do*. Activities may be divided into as many parts as necessary and according to the abilities of the child in question. In this way objectives are planned which have a successful outcome; this ensures that the child is motivated by his success, his parents are encouraged by it and are motivated to participate in helping their child solve his problems.

The system may be used with any type of problem beginning with those at a very basic level, such as learning to look at an object sufficiently long to discern its qualities, increasing range of movement of a rheumatoid joint or learning to cut with scissors along progressively narrower lines.

With this method it is possible to make both long- and short-term plans for a child, to analyse aims and divide them into stages which are realistic for a particular child and provide him and his family with attainable goals. Success leads to increased motivation and the written analysis provides proof of progress and a record of the speed of the progress which will be taken into account when making further plans (Hong, Hill and Blundy, 1986).

'No man is an island', neither is any child. Those who have problems bring those problems to their family. The handicapped child creates a handicapped family. The occupational therapist must not think in terms of upper limb function, the development of play or visuoperceptual skills; she must consider the whole child within his family as one unit and within that unit a number of problems exist in which she will play a part defining and solving.

For the child with continuing impairment, his assessment and subsequent treatment plan is not a once and for all procedure. Reassessments will be necessary and plans will need to be consistently amended. The success of this progression will depend, to a large extent, on effective record keeping.

In 1956, Dr Lawrence Weed began work on problem orientated medical records (POMR). His system has been applied to many areas of medicine and it can be profitably adapted to the needs of those working in paediatrics. It consists of four elements.

1. The data base which consists of all the subjective and objective information which has been gathered about the child.
2. The list of problems affecting the child and his family. Each problem is given a number by which it is referred to throughout the child's records.
3. Initial plans which are drawn up to solve each problem. These will include therapeutic aims and general and specific behavioural objectives for the child.
4. Progress notes which will relate to specific problems and their behavioural objectives. These notes will provide indications of the need for further assessment and amendments of treatment plans, aims and behavioural objectives.

Case note

Graham who suffers from cerebral palsy of diplegic type was referred for occupational therapy soon after he began school.

Date base

1. First child of healthy parents. No problems during the perinatal period.
2. Diplegia was diagnosed at 6 months. First independent steps at three years. Has attended for physiotherapy until the present.
3. He has been under speech therapy review since the age of three because of slight delay in the development of comprehensive and expressive language.
4. His parents gave the following history:
   (a) In addition to the delay in beginning to walk he has had difficulty learning to dress himself and often refuses to try to do so especially on school mornings when time is short.
   (b) He is rather a messy eater: he uses a spoon or a fork but cannot manage a knife and fork. Left to his own devices he prefers to finger feed.
   (c) He enjoys playing with cars and other wheeled toys rather than drawing, colouring or jigsaws.
   (d) He tends to flit from toy to toy, playing with them in a non-specific way.
4. His teachers described the following problems:
   (a) Disruptive behaviour in the classroom.
   (b) Inability to concentrate for more than a few seconds without close adult supervision.
   (c) Complete lack of interest in any activity which requires precise hand skills and close hand-eye co-ordination.

(d) Frequent temper tantrums particularly when his wishes were frustrated.

5. His occupational therapist found it difficult to engage his attention for more than three or four minutes with a single activity. He attempted to divert attention from the task in hand if it was unfamiliar to him by sweeping equipment off the table, leaving his chair and running round the room and touching equipment when he had been forbidden to do so.

(a) Building with 2.5 cm bricks indicated that his finger-thumb grip was imprecise. He had a slight tremor which produced inaccurate placement. His release of the bricks was not as finely graded as would be expected in a five-year-old child. He was unable to build three steps with six bricks even after several demonstrations.

(b) He was able to match colours and select red and yellow when they were named. He was unable to name any colours.

(c) He drew vertical and horizontal lines, a circle and a cross. His drawing of a square was composed of four separate lines. His drawing of a human figure consisted of a head with features and legs. It scored 4.25 years on the Goodenough 'Draw-a-Man' Test. He was not happy with any drawing activity.

(d) He took 80 seconds to complete the Goddard formboard. There was some trial and error and difficulty aligning the star and cross shapes with the inset.

(e) He took 60 seconds to place ten pegs in a pegboard. He used an imprecise right-handed finger-thumb grip.

(f) He snipped paper with scissors but was unable to cut along a line or cut along the outline of a simple shape.

Problems

1. Poor concentration and short attention span.
2. Inability to dress independently.
3. Inability to use a knife and fork.
4. Delayed fine motor skills.
   (a) Poor pencil skills.
   (b) Poor scissor skills.
5. Disruptive behaviour in school.

Initial plans

Graham was being treated at home and in school as a five year old yet his skills had clearly not reached this level. His poor concentration and short attention span were felt to be due to unrealistic goals

being set for him which resulted in frequent failure and hence lack of motivation. The first aim of occupational therapy was therefore to set appropriate tasks for him in order to:
1. Motivate him by ensuring he would be successful.
2. Gain his confidence by providing tasks within his capabilities.
3. Demonstrate to his parents the type of activities which were suitable to his developmental level.
4. Maintain his concentration over increasing periods of time by presenting only the equipment necessary for the current activity and having the rest of the room clear of distractions.

After gaining Graham's confidence therapy will proceed towards the solution of his other problems.

Behavioural objectives

1. (a) Graham will 'drive' a small car along a wide straight road which has been drawn for him on a floor chalkboard.
   (b) He will 'drive' a small car along curved roads and subsequently those with 90 degree angles. (Thus also working towards the solution of problem 4.)
   (c) He will make pictures by scribbling inside stencils of familiar objects such as a house, a lorry, an aeroplane. Where large areas are to be covered both he and his therapist will engage in the activity.
   (d) He will sort Froebel animals by colour.
2. (a) He will choose clothes from a dressing-up box of easily put on clothes and dress up in them. He will take part in this activity in front of a mirror.
   (b) With his occupational therapist he will help to undress himself before he has physiotherapy.
   (c) He will dress with the help of his occupational therapist after physiotherapy sessions. At first he will only be asked to complete putting on a garment, pulling down a vest or adjusting the top of a sock. He will gradually contribute more to dressing himself but he will never be asked to attempt garments which are obviously beyond his abilities. His therapist will use 'backward chaining' — teaching the end of a task first so that Graham has the satisfaction of completion and gradually moving towards the beginning of the task until he can complete it independently.
3. He will eat his lunch at the clinic and try out a variety of spoons and forks. He will hold one implement in each hand. He will choose which implement to use to carry his food to his mouth.
4. (a) He will draw with a pencil to which a triangular pencil grip has been fitted.

(b) He will draw circles by drawing inside a stencil. Later he will draw other shapes in this way.
(c) He will use these stencilled shapes to make houses, faces, etc.

5. (a) He will use scissors to snip pieces off strips of thin card 2 cm wide. At first his therapist will hold the card and later he will hold it himself — a two-handed activity.
(b) He will cut these strips of card along 5 mm wide guide lines. As his cutting becomes more accurate he will cut along narrower lines.
(c) He will cut out straight sided shapes.

Progress notes

1st Session. Enjoyed taking clothes from the dressing-up box, tried to put on cowboy waistcoat, could not find second armhole and he had put it on upsidedown. Abandoned it when he was not successful. Drove car along a wide chalked road, but he became uninterested when a narrower road was drawn. Mother counselled about choosing clothes which are easy to put on without difficult fastenings.

2nd Session. Graham was eager to try the same activities again. After repeating the activities of the previous session, he became boisterous when new activities were suggested. Snipped narrow strips of paper with scissors. He enjoyed drawing horizontal lines between prepared stimulus lines but lost interest when the stimulus lines were narrowed as it required increased accuracy from him. His mother is very concerned about his behaviour in school. School visit to be arranged.

3rd Session. School visit. His teachers are very concerned about his disruptive behaviour. Observation of his class suggested that the overall level was too high for Graham. After discussion of his developmental level, his teachers agreed to work out an appropriate scheme of work for him.

4th Session. Graham is calmer and less apprehensive about attempting new activities. His mother reports that he is happier at school and more willing to talk about what he has been doing. After drawing several squares with a stencil, he drew one free-hand and was very pleased with his success. Dressed in tee shirt and shoes with Velcro fastenings he dressed himself with minimal help after his session with the physiotherapist.

After ten treatment sessions, Graham was co-operative and happy to try new activities. His behavioural objectives were amended to include fastening buttons and buckles, learning to use a knife and fork and a programme to learn how to form letters.

The writing of such records ensures that all problems are considered and that all those dealing with the child are aware of them. They ensure that all that is written down is meaningful and refers to a specific problem. At all times the occupational therapist is giving a professional opinion. The records make it possible to assess the effectiveness of a particular treatment for a child. Because information is recorded in a uniform manner it will be suitable for computerisation and for clinical research purposes. This last point is of great importance: paediatrics is a comparatively new area of occupational therapy and if it is to develop and be of proven value it must be objectively proved to be effective (Mosey, 1981). Only by research can the most effective modes of treatment be discovered and used for the benefit of the child with impairment and his family.

References

Alston, J. and Taylor, J. (1984) *Handwriting File*. L.D.A., Wisbech

Bishop, D.V.M. (1980) Handedness, Clumsiness and Cognitive Ability. *Developmental Medicine and Child Neurology*, 22, 569–79

Blakemore, C. (1977) *Mechanics of the Mind*. Cambridge University Press, Cambridge, pp. 1–4

Bobath, K. (1966) *The Motor Deficit in Patients with Cerebral Palsy*. Medical, Educational and Information Unit of the Spastics Society in Association with Heinemann Medical Boks, London, pp. 30–2

British Association of Occupational Therapists, Way Ahead Working Party (1982) *The Way Ahead*. British Association of Occupational Therapy, London, p. 13

British Orthoptic Society (1979) *Glossary of Terms Used in Orthoptic Practice in the United Kingdom*. The British Orthoptic Society, Manchester

Butts, P.A. (1980) Understanding the Nursing Process. In J. Robinson (ed.), *Documenting Patient Care Responsibility*. Intermed Communications, Pennsylvania, p. 16

Clark, M.M. (1970) *Reading Difficulties in Schools*. Penguin Books, London, pp. 45–9

Corso, J.F. (1967) *The Experimental Psychology of Sensory Behaviour*. Holt, Rinehart and Winston, New York, pp. 148–51, 305–12

Cotton, E. (1984) Integration of disciplines in the treatment and education of children with cerebral palsy. In S. Levitt (ed.), *Paediatric Developmental Therapy*. Blackwell Scientific Publications, Oxford, pp. 249–54

Curzon, L.B. (1980) *Teaching in Further Education*, 2nd edn. Cassell, London, pp. 7, 220–2

Dreier, S. (1980) Principal goals of occupational therapy for visually handicapped infants and toddlers. In R. Bruckner and B. Gloof (eds), *Rehabilitation of the Visually Disabled and the Blind at Different Ages*. Hans Huber, Bern. pp. 28–40

Enstrom, E.A. (1962) The extent of the use of the left hand in handwriting. *Journal of Educational Research*, 55, 234–5

Finnie, N.R. (1974) *Handling the Young Cerebral Palsied Child at Home*, 2nd edn. Heinemann Medical Books, London

Fisch, L. (1969) Hearing Loss and Cerebral Palsy. In S. Blencoe (ed.), *Cerebral Palsy and the Young Child*. E & S Livingstone, Edinburgh, pp. 50, 55

Foley, J. (1969) Associated Disorders. In S. Blencoe (ed.), *Cerebral Palsy and the Young Child*. E & S Livingstone, Edinburgh, pp. 42–3

Francis-Williams, J. (1970) *Children with Specific Learning Difficulties*. Pergamon Press, Oxford, pp. 142–66

Fraser, B.C. (1980) The meaning of handicap in children. *Child: Care, Health and Development*, 6, 83–91

Freeman, P. (1975) *Understanding the Deaf/Blind Child*. Heinemann Medical Books, London, p. 63

Geddes, D. (1976) *Show Me How, a Workbook for Teaching Children with Learning Disabilities*. The Permanent Press, Los Angeles, pp. 63–4, 89–94

Goad, M. (1977) A picture approach to typewriting. *Special Education*, 4, 14–16

Harpin, P. (1981) *With a Little Help*. Vol. 1 Introduction and adaptations. Vol. 2 Bedroom and clothing. Vol. 3 Bathroom. Vol. 4 Household and Seating. Vol. 5 Communication. Vol. 6 Mobility. Vol. 7 Leisure. Vol. 8 Index. The Muscular Dystrophy Group of Great Britain, London

Heddell, T. (1985) *With a Little Help from the Chip*. British Broadcasting Corporation, London, pp. 15–24, 25–8

Holgate, L. (1985) *Young People with Spina Bifida and/or Hydrocephalus — Learning and Development*. ASBAH, London, p. 11–13

Hong, C.S., Hill, J. and Blundy, C. (1986) Using aims and objectives in the Multidisciplinary team. *British Journal of Occupational Therapy*, 49, 100–2

Hosking, G. (1982) *An Introduction to Paediatric Neurology*. Faber and Faber, London, pp. 83–7

Illingworth, R.S. (1980) *The Development of the Infant and Young Child: Normal and Abnormal*. Churchill Livingstone, Edinburgh, pp. 140, 234

Illingworth, R. and Illingworth, C. (1984) *Babies and Young Children. A Guide for Parents*, 7th edn. Churchill Livingstone, Edinburgh, pp. 100–19

Kashani, J.H. (1986) Self-esteem of handicapped children and adolescents. *Developmental Medicine and Child Neurology*, 28, 81–3

Kephart, N.C. (1960) *The Slow Learner in the Classroom*. Chas. E. Merrill Books, Ohio

Kinsbourne, M. (1968) Developmental Gerstmann Syndrome. *Paediatric Clinics of North America*, 15, 771–8

Levy, J. and Reid, M. (1976) Variations in writing posture and cerebral organisation. *Science*, 194, 337–9

Lyle, J.G. and Johnson, E.G. (1976) Development of lateral consistency and its relation to reading and reversals perceptual and motor skills, 43, 695–8

McCarthy, G.T. (1984) *The Physically Handicapped Child*. Faber and Faber, London, pp. 175–8

Montessori, M. (1965) *Dr Montesorri's Own Handbook*. Schocken Book, New York, pp. 49–123

Mosey, A.C. (1981) *Occupational Therapy: Configuration of a Profession*. Raven Press, New York, p. 41–5

Nathan, J. (1969) *The Nervous System*. Penguin Books, London, pp. 81–7, 309

Newton, M. and Thompson, M. (1974) *Dyslexia: a Guide to Teaching*. The University of Aston, Birmingham, pp. 21–2

Newton, M. and Thompson, M. (1976) *Aston Index*. L.D.A., Wisbech

Penso, D. (1981) Remediation built on trust. *Remedial Therapist*, 3, 22

Penso, D. (1983) Some are born lefthanded. *Remedial Therapist*, 5, 5

Pritchard, G.C. (1969) Assessment of vision in young children with cerebral palsy. In S. Blencoe (ed.), *Cerebral Palsy and the Young Child*. E & S Livingstone, Edinburgh, pp. 60–1

Rockey, J. and Nelham, R.L. (1984) Seating for the chairbound child. In G.T. McCarthy (ed.), *The Physically Handicapped Child*. Faber and Faber, London

Sheridan, M.D. (1968) *Manuals of Instruction for STYCAR Test of Vision and Hearing*. NFER-Nelson, Windsor

Sheridan, M.D. (1975) *From Birth to Five Years*. NFER-Nelson, Windsor

Sinclair, D. (1969) *Human Growth After Birth*. Oxford University Press, Oxford, pp. 89–107

Standing, E.M. (1957) *Maria Montesorri Her Life and Work*. The New American Library, New York, pp. 89–228

Taft, L.T. (1972) Are we handicapping the handicapped? *Developmental Medicine and Child Neurology*, 14, 703–4

Touwen, B.C.L. (1972) Laterality and dominance. *Developmental Medicine and Child Neurology*, 14, 747–55

Vasey, E.K. (1980) Documenting patient care. In J. Robinson (ed.), *Documenting Patient Care Responsibiity*. Intermed Communications, Pennsylvania, p. 27

Vernon, P.E. (1960) *Intelligence and Attainment Tests*. University of London Press, London, pp. 31, 45–8

Vernon, M.D. (1971) *The Psychology of Perception*. Penguin Books, London, pp. 20, 21–2, 43, 189

Walker, M. (1985) *The Makaton Vocabulary Development Project*. Camberley, Surrey

Wendon, L. (1973) *The Pictogram System*. Pictogram Supplies, Cambridge

Williams, M. (1970) *Brain Damage and the Mind*. Penguin Books, London, pp. 15–32

Wood, Philip, H.N. (1980) Appreciating the consequences of disease: the international classification of impairments, disabilities and handicaps. *WHO Chronicle*, 34, 376–380

Ziviani, J. (1982) Children's prehension while writing: a pilot study. *British Journal of Occupational Therapy*, 45, 306–7

Further Reading

Allin, R.E. and Lawton, D.S. (1977) *The Management of Juvenile Chronic Polyarthritis*. ACPC Publications, Crawley

Alston, J. (1985) Brittle bones: a handicap with special occupational therapy needs. *British Journal of Occupational Therapy*, 48, 103–5

Ayres, A.J. (1974) *The development of Sensory Integration Theory and Practice*. Kendall/Hunt Publishing Company, Iowa

Bartram, G.E. (1973) *Not Yet Five*. Creative Learning, Harlow

Bayes, K. and Francklins, S. (1971) *Designing for the Handicapped*. George Godwin, London

Bishop, D.V.M. (1984) Using non-preferred hand skill to investigate pathological left-handedness in an unselected population. *Developmental Medicine and Child Neurology*, 214–26

Blissymbolics Communication Foundation (1975) *Syntax Supplement No. 1 Dictionary*. Toronto

Burr, L. (1980) Use of vision in the function of hand eye co-ordination. *British Journal of Occupational Therapy* 43, 59–63

Calnan, J. (1984) *Coping with Research. The Complete Guide for Beginners*. Heinemann Medical Books, London

Carr, J. (1980) *Helping your Handicapped Child: A Step-by-step Guide to Everyday Problems*. Penguin Books, London

Clark, M.M. (1974) *Teaching Left-handed Children*. Hodder & Stoughton, Sevenoaks

Craft, A.W. (1985) Arthritis in children. Paediatric Symposium. *British Journal of Hospital Medicine*, April, 188–94

Cratty, B.J. (1973) *Teaching Motor Skills*. Prentice-Hall, New Jersey

Cunningham, C. (1982) *Down's Syndrome: An Introduction for Parents* (Human Horizons Series). Souvenir Press, London

Cunningham, C. and Davis, H. (1985) *Working with Parents: Frameworks for Collaboration*. Open University Press, Milton Keynes

Deacon, J.J. (1974) *Tongue Tied. Fifty Years of Friendship in a Subnormality Hospital*. National Society for Mentally Handicapped Children, London

Downey, J.A. and Low, N.L. (1982) *The Child with Disabling Illness*. Raven Press, New York

Eysenck, H.J. (1965) *Fact and Fiction in Psychology*. Penguin Books, London

Fahn, S. (1972) Differential Diagnosis of Tremors. *Medical Clinics of North America*, 56, 1363–75

Farnham-Diggory, S. (1978) *Learning Disabilities*. Fontana Open Books, London

Firth, M.A. and Wilkinson, E.J. (1983) Problems reported by parents of boys suffering from duchenne muscular dystrophy. *British Journal of Occupational Therapy*, 46, 306–62

Furneaux, B. (1969) *The Special Child*. Penguin Books, London

George, S.J. and Hart, B. (1983) *Physical Education for Handicapped Children*. Souvenir Press, London

Gloyn, S. and Frobisher, B. (1975) *Teaching Basic Skills to Infants*. Ward Lock, London

Gordon, N. and McKinlay, I. (1980) *Helping Clumsy Children*. Churchill Livingstone, Edinburgh

Grimley, A.M.D. and McKinlay, I.A. (1977) *The Clumsy Child*. ACPC Publications, Crawley

Hall, D.M.B. (1984) *The Child with a Handicap*. Blackwell Scientific Publications, Oxford

Hamilton, A.M. and Shah, S.K. (1984) Physical hand function with spina bifida myelomeningocele. *British Journal of Occupational Therapy*, 47, 147–50

Hartrick, J. (undated) *Equipment to Make — A Guide for Parents with a Child who has a Physical Disability*. Health Commission of Victoria, Australia

Haskell, S.H., Barrett, E.K. and Taylor, H. (1977) *The Education of Motor and Neurologically Handicapped Children*. Croom Helm, London

Hawkridge, D., Vincent, T. and Hales, G. (1983) *New Information Technology in the Education of Disabled Children and Adults*. Croom Helm, London

Holt, J. (1967) *How Children Learn*. Penguin Books, London

Holt, K.S. (1977) *Developmental Paediatrics. Perspectives and Practice* (Postgraduate Paediatric Series). Butterworths, London

Hong, C.S. (1985) The Bobath approach and its application in occupational therapy for children with cerebral palsy. *British Journal of Occupational Therapy*, 48, 4–7

Jones, E.G. (1973) *Children Growing Up*. Penguin Books, London

Josefowicz, A. (1980) Preparing the young handicapped child for school. *British Journal of Occupational Therapy*, 43, 230–2

Leigh, G. (1983) *All about Twins. A Handbook for Parents*. Routledge and Kegan Paul, London

Levitt, S. (1984) *Paediatric Developmental Therapy*. Blackwell Scientific Publications, Oxford

Little, D.E. and Carnevali, D.L. (1976) *Nurse Care Planning*. J.B. Lippincott, New York

Pitt, N. (1975) Typing for the disabled child. *British Journal of Occupational Therapy*, 38, 132–4

Richardson, N.K. (1959) *Type With One Hand*. South Western Publishing Company, New York

Robinson, J. (1980) *Documenting Patient Care Responsibility* (Nursing Skillbook Series). Intermed Communications, Pennsylvania

Rodger, J. and Johnson, G.R. (1982) Moulded seating: techniques of assessment, positioning and casting. *British Journal of Occupational Therapy*, 45, 23–5

Russell, P. (1984) *The Wheelchair Child*. Souvenir Press, London

Sassoon, R. (1983) *The Practical Guide to Children's Handwriting*. Thames and Hudson, London

Turner, A. (1981) *The Practice of Occupational Therapy*. Churchill Livingstone, Edinburgh

Valentine, C.W. (1956) *The Normal Child and Some of His Abnormalities*. Penguin Books, London

Varma, V.P. (1984) *Anxiety in Children*. Croom Helm, London

Vicker, B.A. (1974) *Nonoral Communication System Project 1964–1973*. Campus Stores, Iowa

Walsh, S.R. and Lolzberg, R. (1981) *Understanding and Educating the Deaf/Blind/Severely and Profoundly Handicapped. An International Perspective*. Charles C. Thomas, Illinois

Webster, J.G., Cook, A.M., Tomkins, W.J. and Vanderheiden, G.C. (1984) *Electronic Devices for Rehabilitation*. Chapman and Hall, London

Index